The MRCGP S

T. A. I. Bouchier Hayes
John Fry
Eric Gambrill
Alistair Moulds
K. Young

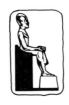

Update Books

The MRCGP Study Book

Tests and self-assessment exercises devised by MRCGP examiners for those preparing for the exam.

by

Lt. Colonel T.A.I. Bouchier Hayes, LAH, FRCGP, DRCOG, is the Trainer in General Practice at the Royal Military Academy, Sandhurst. He was responsible until recently for organising the Army's MRCGP courses for the Services.

John Fry, OBE, MD, FRCS, FRCGP, is a General Practitioner in Beckenham, Kent. He is an Examiner for the MRCGP and was Chairman of the Board of Censors.

Eric Gambrill, MB, BS, FRCGP, D.OBST. RCOG, is a General Practitioner in Crawley, Sussex, and Course Organiser of the Crawley Vocational Training Scheme. He is an Examiner for the MRCGP and was Secretary of the Board of Censors.

Alistair Moulds, MB, CH.B, MRCGP, D.OBST. RCOG, is a General Practitioner in Basildon, Essex. He is involved in the organisation of MRCGP courses.

Col. K. Young, OBE, MB, B.CH, FRCGP, DTM & H, DPH, is Adviser in General Practice to the Director General Army Medical Services based at Millbank. He is a College Examiner and was a member of the Board of Censors. he is also a member of the Armed Services General Practice Approval Board, the joint Committee on Postgraduate Training for General Practice, the Defence Medical Services General Practice Specialty Board, and the Conference of Postgraduate Advisers in General Practice of the Universities of the United Kingdom.

1981 Update Books   London - Dordrecht - Boston

Available in the UK and Eire from:
Update Books Ltd.,
33–34 Alfred Place, London WC1E 7DP, England.

Available in the USA and Canada from:
Kluwer Boston Inc.,
Lincoln Building, 160 Old Derby St., Hingham, Mass. 02043, USA.

Available in the rest of the world from:
Kluwer Academic Publications Group,
Distribution Centre, PO Box 322, 3300 AH Dordrecht, The Netherlands.

British Library Cataloguing in Publication Data

The MRCGP study book.
  1. Medicine – Great Britain – Examinations
  I. Bouchier-Hayes, T
  610'.76   R837.E9

  ISBN 0-906141-13-3

ISBN 0 906141 31 1 (Paperback) ISBN 0 906141 13 3 (Hardback)

Typeset and produced by:
R. James Hall Typesetting & Book Production Services
Harpenden, England
Typeface: IBM Press Roman 10pt on 11
Printed in Great Britain by
Redwood Burn Limited, Trowbridge
and bound by Pegasus Bookbinding, Melksham

Contents

Foreword

The Membership examination of the Royal College of General Practitioners has evolved and matured as a seal and a test on completion of vocational training. More than 1000 candidates are taking the examination each year and an increasing majority are trainees who have completed their three-year training period.

The whole concept and philosophy of the MRCGP has been questioned by critical cynics who refuse to accept general practice as a field of medical practice worthy of recognition as a specialty with its own core of knowledge, skills and expertise and with its own special epidemiology, pathology, clinical presentations and management. These cynical critics are being answered by the growth of the examination and its recognition within the profession as an important and necessary goal to be achieved. The MRCGP exam has arrived, it is here to stay and it will continue to grow and evolve.

The exam is no easy obstacle to negotiate. It has a regular failure rate of 1 in 3 and it requires special preparation and study of its examinees if they are to understand its aims, contents and methods. It must not be assumed that even the brightest trainee can walk off the street, enter the examination hall and be confident of passing. It requires a few months of careful and guided preparation.

The objectives of this book are to help the MRCGP candidate, and his tutors, to prepare for the exam. It is no comprehensive text book and it is no cookbook of tests and checks. Rather it describes the examination and its parts and analyses its objectives. The book provides examples of questions and the ways in which they are set out and it suggests ways in which they might be answered.

Some multiple choice questions have been adapted from questions originally composed by A. J. Moulds for *Doctor* magazine's "Ten Minute Test" and we should like to thank the editorial staff and readers of *Doctor* for the helpful and constructive criticisms that they have made in the past.

The Study Book is designed to supplement the advice given in *The MRCGP Examination – A Comprehensive Guide to Preparation and Passing* by A. J. Moulds, T. A. I. Bouchier Hayes and K. Young, published by MTP Press Limited. We should like to thank Mr David Bloomer, Managing Director of MTP, for kindly allowing these authors to be involved in both projects.

The authors are past and present examiners and tutors concerned in organising courses for the exam. They are well aware of the examiners' expectations and the candidates' problems.

This book is dedicated to future generations of MRCGP candidates in the conviction that their decision to become good general practitioners is welcome and praiseworthy and that their desire to become members of the Royal College of General Practitioners is a right and proper sign of their striving for high standards of care and practice.

John Fry
London, 1981

Introduction

Why the Exam?

Britain has more examinations for medical qualifications and for postgraduate qualifications than any other country. Nowhere else in the world can a medically registered person place so many letters after his name! Attempts have been made to scale down the numbers of qualifications and the examinations necessary to achieve them. So why is there an examination for general practice?

Until World War II the objective of our undergraduate medical education was to produce a 'safe doctor' who could immediately go into general practice without any further training or experience. Many general practitioners did just this. They went through a five-year undergraduate programme, gained their degrees, or, more usually then, the conjoint diplomas, borrowed money, bought their practices and set up as single-handed general practitioners, where they stayed in medical isolation for the remainder of their professional lives. Many became good general practitioners, after some years spent developing their skills at the expense of their patients!

After World War II, and with the introduction of the National Health Service, it became clear that some preparation and tutelage for general practice was necessary. The trainee assistant scheme was set up. A general practitioner applied to be approved as a trainer and, if accepted, was allowed to employ a trainee assistant for a year. No attempt was made to provide any formal teaching and there were no official training programmes. There was no assessment at the end of the year and almost no supervision of the trainer.

With the foundation of the College of General Practitioners in 1952 and the re-awakening of self-confidence, it became clear that if general practice was to develop and progress it had to become a specialty in its own right. As a specialty it had to have its own training programme, and as an essential part of such a programme there had to be some form of assessment.

After 10 years the College foundations became firm enough for the founders to realise that entry into its membership should involve more than just paying a token club entry and annual membership fees. As its sister colleges had done, the College of General Practitioners, amidst considerable internal and external opposition, decided to introduce an examination as a condition of entry.

The College Examination

After beginning in the 1960s with a handful of candidates, the MRCGP exam is now taken by more than 1,200 candidates each year at two annual examination sessions.

The MRCGP exam has developed progressively into the end-point for the three-year vocational training programme. The proportion of more senior established prac-

1

titioners taking the exam is decreasing and the proportion of trainees is increasing. The present ratio is around 35:65.

From its earliest days the MRCGP exam has been a combination of written papers and orals. Periodic consideration has been given to introducing clinical cases, either of 'real' patients or of actors, but the methodology has been too difficult and the costs too high.

The exam consists of two stages for those who stay the whole course. First, there is a day of papers for all candidates. Second, an invitation to attend for an oral examination is sent to those candidates whose marks in the papers are considered high enough to give them a chance of reaching the pass mark in the orals.

The objective of the examination is to test the candidate's knowledge and understanding of the basic content of general practice conditions and situations, to test his attitude to his work and to test his understanding of the problems of organisation within a practice, of promoting the health of his patients, of preventing disease and of coordinating logical hospital, community and practice services for his patients.

The MRCGP exam is no walk-over. It is a challenging test and a stressful experience for all candidates. The pass rates have ranged at various times from 55 per cent to almost 75 per cent.

It is rash and foolhardy to sit the examination without careful preparation and reading.

The Format

The current format of the MRCGP exam will now be described. Each part is dealt with in detail later in this book.

Multiple Choice Questions (MCQ)

These questions are set by the examiners to test knowledge and factual recall. They are specifically related to general practice and attempt to cover a large part of the field.

Modified Essay Question (MEQ)

This form of test has been specially developed for the MRCGP. The question consists of an extended case history from general practice.

During the course of the case a number of events or situations occur and the candidate is asked a series of questions relating to them. These situations may be clinical but they may also be organisational, attitudinal, social or personal involving the practitioner, the patient and the family.

The MEQ is the closest attempt to a clinical test in the exam and requires considerable thought and experience on the part of the candidate to achieve high marks.

Traditional Essay Questions (TEQ)

This paper contains the more traditional essay questions. Some of these questions may deal with general issues relating to health care and its organisation; others may cover clinical and therapeutic matters and there may be still more topics introduced at any time.

The Orals

Candidates taking the oral part of the exam are interviewed by two pairs of examiners. The first pair will base their questions on the candidate's practice and his own cases in his Log Diary. The second pair may pose any questions but they tend to be based on the examiner's own clinical material and include problems of personal, family and social management.

The orals give the examiners their only chance to meet the candidates face to face and offer the candidates a chance to impress by their manner, professional approach and knowledge.

Marking

The MRCGP exam is a professionally run exercise. It is prepared by examiners who have become expert in each of the various parts.

Each part and its questions are carefully thought out and the value of the marks awarded for each part carefully decided upon.

The marking of papers is carried out by all the examiners and each paper is assessed by at least two examiners. If their marks vary greatly then the paper is re-examined and assessed further.

Considerable efforts are made to see that the marking is fair and accurate.

Multiple Choice Questions or MCQ

The MCQ is one of the five major parts of the MRCGP examination and, as such, is worth one-fifth of the total examination marks. In the near future it may become separated from the rest of the exam to be reconstituted as MRCGP part one, providing a barrier which candidates have to pass in order to be allowed to sit the rest of the exam at a later date. Regardless of changes in the timings of the parts of the exam the essential features of the MCQ will remain unchanged and the advice given here will still apply. While the exam as a whole seeks to test attitudes, problem-solving abilities, interview skills and factual knowledge, it is only the last of these that is tested by the MCQ.

General Structure of the MCQ Paper

In three hours 90 five-part questions have to be answered. Each question is of the multiple true/false variety and has a 'stem' statement followed by the five items or completions requiring true/false/don't know answers. The 'stem' statement is considered with each item in turn and, when answering, you should disregard all the other items in that question as they have nothing to do with the one you are concentrating on. A total of 450 answers have to be given in the three hours allotted but, although this may seem like a tall order, the time allowed is more than adequate.

An example of a typical question is:

Potassium retaining diuretics include (*'Stem'*)

  A Amiloride

  B Chlorthalidone

  C Bumetanide

  D Spironolactone

  E Frusemide
(5 'items' or 'completions')

The answer in this case is true, false, false, true, false but it is important to note that any combination of true and false may occur and there is nothing to prevent all items being true or, equally, all items being false.

The proportion of the 90 questions devoted to the different areas of general practice knowledge is obviously important as it should influence the time you spend revising each subject. Currently the College say the breakdown of questions is as shown below:

General medicine	20	questions
Psychiatry	18	"
Obstetrics and gynaecology	12	"
Therapeutics	10	"
Paediatrics	10	"
Surgical diagnosis	5	"
Ear, nose and throat Ophthalmology Dermatology	10	"
Community medicine	5	"

In fact, it appears recently that paediatrics and therapeutics questions have markedly increased in number at the expense of psychiatry and obstetrics questions. Whatever the actual breakdown among the first five subjects listed may now be, it is fair to note that the second five subjects listed account for only 20 of the 90 questions. Therefore it would be reasonable to spend only a little time on their revision.

The question paper itself is in book form and the answers have to be recorded on separate computer marking or Opscan sheets (you will see this sheet at the beginning of each of the four tests at the end of this chapter).

Each question part has its own true/false/don't know boxes, only one of which has to be filled in with the pencil provided. The computer marks by photoelectric scanning and will select the most heavily shaded box as the given answer. It will also reject papers where no box has been filled in as even a don't know is taken account of in the marking.

This is because the marking system used is a negative one. Therefore:

a correct answer scores	+1
an incorrect answer scores	-1
a don't know scores	0

This is of vital importance as random guessing is heavily penalised and your approach to your answering should take full account of it. To elaborate, using one question as an example:

Live vaccines include

A Pertussis

B Measles

C Poliomyelitis

D Rabies

E BCG

F T T F T would score	5 out of 5
T T T F T would score	3 out of 5
D T T F T would score	4 out of 5
T T T T T would score	1 out of 5
D T T D T would score	3 out of 5
T T T T F would score	-1 out of 5

Complete guessing over a negatively marked paper would give a score of 0 per cent (assuming half were guessed right and half wrong), whereas complete guessing with a non-punitive marking system would give 50 per cent.

In situations where candidates have a reasonable idea of what the correct answer is but are not certain, guessing is no longer random but calculated or inspired. Calculated guessing can improve a candidate's score.

Structure of Questions

Having described the general style of the paper, it is now worth briefly considering the questions themselves as they can sometimes pose problems. Each part of a question should be testing only one item of knowledge and should use words that are easily understood. Testing of English language knowledge is not an aim and stems and items should be unambiguous. Unfortunately some questions which appear clear to nearly everyone can appear ambiguous to someone who may have a far more detailed knowledge of an individual field than the question is trying to get at. The only advice to be offered is that there are no trick questions and that they should all be taken at their face value. If there is genuine doubt in the mind of the candidate then it is probably safest to mark in a don't know.

If a stem or item does cause confusion then the standard computer analysis of the paper will pick it up and produce an amended score for the question and also allow that question to be replaced in the future. Thus the College's bank of questions is continually being refined to produce ever fairer degrees of discrimination between candidates.

Advice

1. Read each question carefully.

2. Remember you are considering the stem and one item together. Disregard the other items in the question as they have nothing to do with the one you are concentrating on.

3. Answer each item as true, false or don't know and make sure your answer is clear and in the correct box.

4, DO NOT GUESS. Questions you genuinely have no idea about mark as don't know and move onto more productive areas. Those that you think you could work out either consider there and then or leave and come back to at the end.

5. Accept questions at face value. Do not look for hidden catches or tricks. The examiner is not trying to confuse you, and the obvious meaning of his statement is the correct one.

6. Depending on your temperament either go through the whole paper filling the questions you are sure of and then come back to the others at the end *or* systematically work your way through the whole paper. The first method has the advantage of ensuring that no questions you could have answered are left over at the end (if you run out of time), although it does require a fair deal of mental agility. It also allows you to add up the number of 'correct' answers you are reasonably sure of and assess whether you need to guess some. (275

correct out of 450 would give a score of 61 per cent, if all were really correct, but it still allows some leeway for error as the passmark is about 55 per cent.)

7. If you have time to spare at the end check you have put down the answers you meant to and ensure that they are in the correct boxes.

Practising MCQ Papers

As well as the four mock tests in this chapter, MCQ tests may be found in:

1. *The Multiple Choice Question in Medicine.* Anderson. London: Pitman, 1976.

2. *The MRCGP Examination (A comprehensive Guide to Preparation and Passing).* Moulds, Bouchier-Hayes, Young. Lancaster: MTP, 1978.

3. *MCQ Tutor for the MRCGP Examination.* Moulds, Bouchier-Hayes. London: Heinemann, 1980.

Hints for Using the Mock Tests in this Book

Four tests, each of 30 questions, follow. They reflect the subject composition of the College exam and should each be done in one hour under exam conditions.

Answers should be filled in on the Opscan sheets provided at each test's start, and self-marking should be strictly based on the negative marking system.

The first test contains a number of technique points (TPs) designed to emphasise aspects of this form of exam.

Any answers that you strongly disagree with should be checked as, although we are not infallible, we have taken considerable care to be correct!

SURNAME	INITIALS

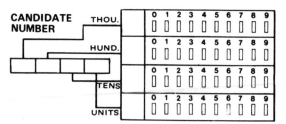

CANDIDATE NUMBER

THOU. 0 1 2 3 4 5 6 7 8 9

HUND. 0 1 2 3 4 5 6 7 8 9

TENS 0 1 2 3 4 5 6 7 8 9

UNITS 0 1 2 3 4 5 6 7 8 9

PAGE No.
1

T means TRUE F means FALSE D means DO NOT KNOW

	1A T F D	1B T F D	1C T F D	1D T F D	1E T F D		2A T F D	2B T F D	2C T F D	2D T F D	2E T F D
1						2					
3	3A	3B	3C	3D	3E	4	4A	4B	4C	4D	4E
5	5A	5B	5C	5D	5E	6	6A	6B	6C	6D	6E
7	7A	7B	7C	7D	7E	8	8A	8B	8C	8D	8E
9	9A	9B	9C	9D	9E	10	10A	10B	10C	10D	10E
11	11A	11B	11C	11D	11E	12	12A	12B	12C	12D	12E
13	13A	13B	13C	13D	13E	14	14A	14B	14C	14D	14E
15	15A	15B	15C	15D	15E	16	16A	16B	16C	16D	16E
17	17A	17B	17C	17D	17E	18	18A	18B	18C	18D	18E
19	19A	19B	19C	19D	19E	20	20A	20B	20C	20D	20E
21	21A	21B	21C	21D	21E	22	22A	22B	22C	22D	22E
23	23A	23B	23C	23D	23E	24	24A	24B	24C	24D	24E
25	25A	25B	25C	25D	25E	26	26A	26B	26C	26D	26E
27	27A	27B	27C	27D	27E	28	28A	28B	28C	28D	28E
29	29A	29B	29C	29D	29E	30	30A	30B	30C	30D	30E

Each cell contains T F D answer markers.

Time allowed – one hour

All questions must be answered by filling in the true/false or don't know boxes on the computer marking sheet.

1 Tolbutamide

  A Should only be given once daily.

  B Is only effective when some residual beta cell activity is present.

  C Does not cause hypoglycaemia as a side effect.

  D May cause facial flushing after drinking alcohol.

  E Should be preferred to a biguanide in the management of an obese diabetic.

TP Part E tells you (if you did not already know) that tolbutamide is a sulphonylurea. In general you will not get information from one question part to help you with another. Remember to consider the stem statement and each item or completion individually to give the question you have to answer.

2 Reiter's syndrome

  A Always occurs in men.

  B In the majority of cases initially presents with conjunctivitis.

  C May follow bacillary dysentery.

  D Arthritis is a monoarthritis.

  E Responds well to penicillin therapy.

3 With rubella it is correct to say

  A The majority of women of childbearing age are immune.

  B Serum antibodies have a low order of protection against reinfection.

  C Congenitally infected infants cannot synthesize their own rubella antibody.

  D Once the rash clears the patient is no longer infectious.

  E Subclinical infection in early pregnancy is as dangerous to the fetus as clinical infection.

4 Characteristic features of predominantly aggressive psychopaths include

  A History of a happy childhood.

  B Sustained violent conduct.

  C Undue sensitivity to the feelings of others.

  D An abnormal EEG.

  E Complete lack of insight.

5 The prostate gland

  A Is purely a sexual organ.

  B If removed leads to permanent absence of ejaculate in the majority of cases.

  C In early hypertrophy classically gives nocturia at 2 to 3 a.m.

  D Diagnosis of carcinoma is reliably made on history alone.

  E If carcinomatous produces a diagnostic elevation of serum alkaline phosphatase.

6 Cimetidine (Tagamet)

  A Inhibits basal gastric secretion of acid.

  B Is best given between meals.

  C Gives immediate symptomatic relief.

  D Has no known contraindications to its use.

  E May cause diarrhoea.

9

7 ECG signs that may occur in a patient as a result of taking digoxin include

A Depression of the ST segment.
B Increased amplitude of the T waves.
C Coupled ventricular extrasystoles.
D Complete heart block.
E Bradycardia.

TP With this kind of question you either know the answers or you don't. You cannot work them out so *Don't* guess. Remember with negative marking you score -1 for every incorrect answer.

8 In non-accidental injury to children

A The first or last child in a family is more likely to be affected.
B The father is the batterer in the majority of cases.
C Injury is more likely at meal times than the rest of the day.
D Arm and shin bruises are especially suspicious.
E The parents may remove the child from hospital at any time unless a place of safety order has been signed by a magistrate.

9 Ectopic pregnancy

A Accounts for about 7 per cent of maternal deaths in GB.
B In the majority of cases is associated with previous tubal infection.
C Shows an increased incidence in progestogen only pill users.
D Nearly always presents with irregular bleeding followed by pain.
E Is best diagnosed in general practice by bimanual vaginal examination.

10 Psoriasis

A Affects nearly two per cent of the population.

B When it affects the scalp may lead to baldness.
C Arthritis produces a positive rheumatoid factor.
D Involving the genitalia, may safely be treated with dithranol in Lassar's paste.
E Tends to improve during pregnancy.

11 Recognised features of diabetic neuropathy include

A Sudden diplopia.
B Painful priapism.
C Constipation.
D Wasting of the calf muscles.
E Increased lower limb reflexes.

TP A recognised feature is one that has been reported and that is a fact that a candidate would reasonably be expected to know.

12 Gonorrhoea

A Can be diagnosed by the rapid plasma reagin (RPR) test.
B Has the same incidence in GP as primary and secondary syphilis.
C If rectal may present with tenesmus.
D Can readily be diagnosed in women by speculum examination.
E Generally responds well to a single dose of ampicillin 2 g and probenecid 1 g by mouth.

13 Glue ear

A Is the most common cause of hearing loss in children.
B Is characterised by collection of pus in the middle ear.
C Is invariably caused by enlarged adenoids.
D May be treated by the insertion of grommets.

E May eventually lead to sensorineural deafness.

14 With normal development a child should be able to

A Follow a object through 180° (while lying supine) at three months of age.
B Show no head lag at five months.
C Feed self with a biscuit at seven months.
D Creep at eight months.
E Spontaneously join two to three words together to make a sentence at 15 months.

15 Well recognised features of grief reactions include

A Hostility towards others.
B Increased mortality among the bereaved.
C Feelings of guilt.
D Psychosomatic symptoms.
E Resolution within about four to six weeks.

16 Characteristic features of Parkinson's disease include

A Tics.
B Extensor plantar responses.
C Hypotonia.
D Tremor during sleep.
E Increased salivation.

TP A characteristic feature is one which occurs so often as, usually, to be of some diagnostic significance and if not present might lead to doubt being cast on the diagnosis.

17 It is correct to say

A The serum K^+ concentration is a reliable indication of the total body stores of K^+.

B For equivalent diuretic effect frusemide will produce a greater fall in K^+ than a thiazide.
C K^+ supplements have no effect on total body K^+.
D Reduction of salt intake will have no effect on K^+ loss.
E The majority of patients taking diuretics for hypertension or heart failure do not require K^+ replacement therapy.

18 In the management of a case of acute pulmonary oedema

A The foot of the bed should be raised.
B IV aminophylline may cause vomiting.
C Oxygen should only be given at a low concentration.
D IV morphine is immediately effective in helping to relieve dyspnoea.
E IV digoxin is best avoided.

19 Infantile rotavirus gastroenteritis

A Generally occurs in the summer.
B Rarely causes fever.
C Produces loose slimy stools.
D Is best managed by using water with concentrated salt as a rehydration fluid.
E Is helped by the use of antidiarrhoeal agents.

20 Typical features of ulnar nerve compression at the elbow include

A Marked predominance of sensory rather than motor symptoms.
B Normal interossei.
C Weakness of adductor pollicis.
D Slight clawing of the fourth and fifth fingers.
E Wasting of the hypothenar muscles.

TP A typical feature is one that you would expect to be present.

21 Characteristic features of endogenous depression include

A Feelings of passivity.
B Grandiose delusions.
C Nearly always feeling better after a good cry.
D Disturbed time sense.
E Increased duration of dreaming.

22 The combined pill is absolutely contra-indicated if there is a past history of

A Superficial thrombophlebitis.
B Mild hepatitis.
C Fibroadenosis of the breasts.
D Thalassaemia trait.
E Cholestatic jaundice of pregnancy.

23 Under the Misuse of Drugs Act 1971

A Synthetic narcotics are not controlled.
B A prescription for a controlled drug must state the total quantity in words only.
C A locked car is not a 'locked receptacle' for the purposes of the Act.
D If a GP suspects a person of being an addict then he must inform the Home Office within one week.
E The register of controlled drugs that each GP must keep has to be a bound book.

24 Cystic fibrosis

A Has a survival rate of 25 per cent at 10 years.
B Is characteristically associated with anorexia.
C Produces excessive loss of NaCl in sweat.
D Should be suspected in any child with recurrent upper respiratory tract infections.
E Is associated with the development of overt diabetes in the majority of cases.

25 Recognised effects of anticholinergic drugs include

A Pupil constriction.
B Bradycardia.
C Dryness of the mouth.
D Slowing of micturition.
E Bronchial constriction.

26 A 48 year old woman develops jaundice. Features that would suggest it was obstructive in origin include

A Normal coloured stools.
B Urobilinogen in the urine.
C Normal alkaline phosphatase.
D Lowered serum cholesterol.
E Absence of pruritus.

27 Recognised features of delerium tremens include

A Drowsiness.
B Excessive sweating.
C Loss of all desire for alcohol.
D Dilated pupils.
E Fine tremor.

TP Remember the negative marking system. For each answer you get correct, score +1; for each incorrect, score -1; for each don't know, score 0. Complete guessing does not pay.

28 In pregnancy

A Nearly all gravidae show an early fall in the Hb concentration.
B Urinary oestrogens form the basis for routine immunological pregnancy tests.
C Drug passage through the stomach is speeded up.
D Maternal iron deficiency leads to neo-natal iron deficiency.
E Fasting blood sugar levels are greater than in the non-pregnant state.

29 Well recognised features of acute iritis include

    A Conjunctival injection
    B Dilation of the pupil.
    C Absence of photophobia.
    D Posterior synechiae.
    E Keratic precipitates.

30 Ejection systolic murmurs are characteristic of

    A Aortic stenosis.
    B Mitral incompetence.
    C Pulmonary stenosis.
    D Tricuspid incompetence.
    E Ventricular septal defect.

THE ANSWERS TO MCQ TEST 1 BEGIN ON PAGE 31

SURNAME	INITIALS

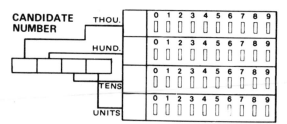

CANDIDATE NUMBER

THOU. 0 1 2 3 4 5 6 7 8 9

HUND. 0 1 2 3 4 5 6 7 8 9

TENS 0 1 2 3 4 5 6 7 8 9

UNITS 0 1 2 3 4 5 6 7 8 9

PAGE No.
1

T means TRUE F means FALSE D means DO NOT KNOW

1	1A	1B	1C	1D	1E		2	2A	2B	2C	2D	2E
	T F D	T F D	T F D	T F D	T F D			T F D	T F D	T F D	T F D	T F D
3	3A	3B	3C	3D	3E		4	4A	4B	4C	4D	4E
	T F D	T F D	T F D	T F D	T F D			T F D	T F D	T F D	T F D	T F D
5	5A	5B	5C	5D	5E		6	6A	6B	6C	6D	6E
	T F D	T F D	T F D	T F D	T F D			T F D	T F D	T F D	T F D	T F D
7	7A	7B	7C	7D	7E		8	8A	8B	8C	8D	8E
	T F D	T F D	T F D	T F D	T F D			T F D	T F D	T F D	T F D	T F D
9	9A	9B	9C	9D	9E		10	10A	10B	10C	10D	10E
	T F D	T F D	T F D	T F D	T F D			T F D	T F D	T F D	T F D	T F D
11	11A	11B	11C	11D	11E		12	12A	12B	12C	12D	12E
	T F D	T F D	T F D	T F D	T F D			T F D	T F D	T F D	T F D	T F D
13	13A	13B	13C	13D	13E		14	14A	14B	14C	14D	14E
	T F D	T F D	T F D	T F D	T F D			T F D	T F D	T F D	T F D	T F D
15	15A	15B	15C	15D	15E		16	16A	16B	16C	16D	16E
	T F D	T F D	T F D	T F D	T F D			T F D	T F D	T F D	T F D	T F D
17	17A	17B	17C	17D	17E		18	18A	18B	18C	18D	18E
	T F D	T F D	T F D	T F D	T F D			T F D	T F D	T F D	T F D	T F D
19	19A	19B	19C	19D	19E		20	20A	20B	20C	20D	20E
	T F D	T F D	T F D	T F D	T F D			T F D	T F D	T F D	T F D	T F D
21	21A	21B	21C	21D	21E		22	22A	22B	22C	22D	22E
	T F D	T F D	T F D	T F D	T F D			T F D	T F D	T F D	T F D	T F D
23	23A	23B	23C	23D	23E		24	24A	24B	24C	24D	24E
	T F D	T F D	T F D	T F D	T F D			T F D	T F D	T F D	T F D	T F D
25	25A	25B	25C	25D	25E		26	26A	26B	26C	26D	26E
	T F D	T F D	T F D	T F D	T F D			T F D	T F D	T F D	T F D	T F D
27	27A	27B	27C	27D	27E		28	28A	28B	28C	28D	28E
	T F D	T F D	T F D	T F D	T F D			T F D	T F D	T F D	T F D	T F D
29	29A	29B	29C	29D	29E		30	30A	30B	30C	30D	30E
	T F D	T F D	T F D	T F D	T F D			T F D	T F D	T F D	T F D	T F D

Time allowed — one hour

All questions must be answered by filling in the true/false or don't know boxes on the computer marking sheet.

1 Recognised side effects of phenytoin therapy include

A Hirsutism
B B_{12} deficiency.
C Gum hyperplasia
D Nystagmus.
E Overbreathing.

2 Characteristic features of polymyalgia rheumatica include

A Sudden onset.
B Severe morning stiffness.
C Polyarthritis.
D Muscle wasting.
E Poor response to high dose oral corticosteroid therapy.

3 Epidemiological studies of headaches have proved that

A Women at all ages suffer more headaches than men.
B Headache prevalence increases with increasing age.
C Migraine sufferers are of higher intelligence than the general population.
D Visual defects are a frequent cause of headaches.
E Mild to moderate hypertension will produce headaches in the majority of cases.

4 Euphoria is a recognised symptom of

A Corticosteroid therapy.
B Multiple sclerosis.
C Psychopathic states.
D A lesion of the parietal lobe.
E A post migraine state.

5 Alopecia areata

A Causes arrest of hair synthesis without destroying the follicles.
B May be an autoimmune disorder.
C Is more common in diabetics.
D Treatment by repeated local injections of triamcinolone will have no adverse effects.
E In the majority of cases hair will regrow spontaneously within three months.

6 It is correct to say that

A Sweating is a constant characteristic of febrile illnesses.
B The recommended time for oral temperature recording is three minutes.
C The normal rectal temperature is 37.3°C.
D The majority of febrile convulsions are without sequelae.
E Pyrexia exists only when the oral temperature is greater than 37.5°C.

7 Nappy rash

A In the majority of cases will be secondarily infected with *Candida* after 72 hours.
B Characteristically spares the skin creases and folds.

15

C Is less likely to occur if the baby wears plastic pants.
D With small pustules indicates *Candida* superinfection.
E May be helped by zinc and castor oil ointment.

8 Metronidazole (Flagyl)

A Is inactive against aerobic organisms.
B Should normally be taken between meals.
C May darken the urine.
D In a single 2 g dose is satisfactory for treatment of trichomonas infestation.
E Patients should be advised to abstain from alcohol while on the drug.

9 In the premenstrual syndrome

A Less than 10 per cent of women of child-bearing age are sufferers.
B Symptoms disappear after hysterectomy.
C The basic problem is most probably a relative excess of progesterone in the second half of the menstrual cycle.
D Diuretic therapy will relieve all symptoms.
E The menstrual chart can be used as a diagnostic tool.

10 Characteristic features of osteoarthrosis of the knee include

A Pain increasing with exercise.
B Prolonged morning stiffness.
C Redness of the joint area.
D Quadriceps wasting.
E Early limping.

11 Recognised features of vertebrobasilar insufficiency include

A Vertigo.
B Dysphasia.
C Drop attacks.
D Glove and stocking anaesthesia.
E Ataxia.

12 Recognised potential hazards of sex hormone replacement therapy include

A Gall bladder disease.
B Cancer of the breast.
C Osteoporosis.
D Endometrial cancer.
E Urogenital atrophy.

13 Laryngeal carcinoma

A Is equally common in females and males.
B Should be suspected when hoarseness persists for more than two weeks.
C Is strongly related to cigarette smoking.
D Has the best prognosis when the tumour is confined to the vocal chord.
E When treated by total laryngectomy sometimes leaves the patient unable to speak normally.

14 In a five month baby signs of dehydration include

A Tachypnoea.
B Increased skin turgor.
C Decreased urinary output.
D Weight loss.
E Bulging anterior fontanelle.

15 Characteristic symptoms of dementia include

A Clouding of consciousness.
B Loss of intelligence.
C Impairment of memory.
D Emotional lability.
E Disorientation for time.

16 In diabetes

A The central diagnostic feature is persistent hyperglycaemia.

B Diagnosis, a random non-fasting blood sugar of greater than 200 mg/dl (11.1 mmol/l) is pathological.
C A patient injecting four marks of 40 strength insulin is getting 16 units of insulin.
D Of maturity onset, renal failure is the most likely cause of death.
E Dot and blot haemorrhages signify proliferative retinopathy.

17 Recognised adverse drug interactions may occur between amitriptyline and

A Alcohol.
B Thyroxine.
C Clonidine.
D Phenytoin.
E Levodopa.

18 There is a recognised association between hydramnios and

A Twin pregnancy.
B First pregnancy.
C Gross fetal abnormality.
D Post partum haemorrhage.
E Prolapse of the cord.

19 In a child with high pyrexia

A The higher the temperature above 40°C (104°F) then the greater the risk of fits.
B Paracetamol has little antipyretic effect.
C Increased fluid intake is only needed if vomiting has occurred.
D Sponging with cold water will invariably decrease the temperature.
E Above 40.5°C (105°F) admission to hospital should be arranged.

20 Well recognised risk factors in suicide include

A Incapacitating physical illness.
B Early dementia.
C Age below 40 years.
D Presence of paranoid delusions.
E Recent retirement.

21 A 49 year old man complains of pain in the right calf after walking 40 to 50 yards but never has pain at rest. Expected findings on clinical examination include

A Absent foot pulses.
B Trophic changes in the skin and toe-nails.
C Pallor of the foot when dependent.
D Positive Holman's sign.
E Varicose veins.

22 In cervical spondylosis

A The C6 and C7 nerve roots are affected in the majority of cases.
B Only sensory symptoms occur.
C Horner's syndrome may occur.
D Spasticity of the lower limbs may develop.
E An immobilizing collar will not relieve nerve root symptoms.

23 Notifiable infectious diseases include

A Tuberculosis.
B Mumps.
C Acute encephalitis.
D Food poisoning.
E Influenza.

24 In Perthes' disease

A Presentation is usually between 3 and 10 years of age.
B Infarction of the proximal femoral epiphysis occurs.
C There is no pain in the hip.
D All haematological investigations are normal.
E The patient develops a limp.

25 Dithranol

A Is effective treatment in acute guttate psoriasis.
B Has no effect on normal skin.
C May be combined with Lassar's paste.
D May stain clothes a purplish colour.
E Is best used initially in high concentrations (1 per cent or more).

26 In an 18-year-old known diabetic in coma the following findings would suggest hypoglycaemia

A Kussmaul breathing.
B Signs of dehydration.
C Profuse sweating.
D Bounding pulse.
E A history of abdominal pain.

27 After eye injury

A Visual acuity should be measured at the outset.
B Pupil dilators may give great relief from pain.
C All chemical burns involving the globe should be referred early for hospital treatment.
D If serious damage has occurred then the GP should carry out as full an examination as possible before referral to hospital.
E A penetrating wound may be indicated by a deformed (oval) pupil.

28 A cervical erosion

A Is an area of cervix denuded of epithelium.
B Will resolve during pregnancy.
C Cannot occur before puberty.
D May cause a discharge.
E Predisposes to cancer of the cervix.

29 Characteristic features of schizophrenia include

A Poor memory for recent events.
B Disharmony between mood and thought.
C Artistic talent.
D Good insight.
E Delusions of guilt.

30 In paroxysmal supraventricular tachycardia

A The pulse rate is about 200 beats per minute.
B The rhythm is completely regular.
C Urina spastica may occur.
D Vagal stimulation may stop the tachycardia abruptly.
E Digoxin is contraindicated.

THE ANSWERS TO MCQ TEST 2 BEGIN ON PAGE 35

SURNAME

INITIALS

CANDIDATE NUMBER

THOU. 0 1 2 3 4 5 6 7 8 9

HUND. 0 1 2 3 4 5 6 7 8 9

TENS 0 1 2 3 4 5 6 7 8 9

UNITS 0 1 2 3 4 5 6 7 8 9

PAGE No.
1

T means **TRUE** **F** means **FALSE** **D** means **DO NOT KNOW**

	A	B	C	D	E
1	1A	1B	1C	1D	1E
2	2A	2B	2C	2D	2E
3	3A	3B	3C	3D	3E
4	4A	4B	4C	4D	4E
5	5A	5B	5C	5D	5E
6	6A	6B	6C	6D	6E
7	7A	7B	7C	7D	7E
8	8A	8B	8C	8D	8E
9	9A	9B	9C	9D	9E
10	10A	10B	10C	10D	10E
11	11A	11B	11C	11D	11E
12	12A	12B	12C	12D	12E
13	13A	13B	13C	13D	13E
14	14A	14B	14C	14D	14E
15	15A	15B	15C	15D	15E
16	16A	16B	16C	16D	16E
17	17A	17B	17C	17D	17E
18	18A	18B	18C	18D	18E
19	19A	19B	19C	19D	19E
20	20A	20B	20C	20D	20E
21	21A	21B	21C	21D	21E
22	22A	22B	22C	22D	22E
23	23A	23B	23C	23D	23E
24	24A	24B	24C	24D	24E
25	25A	25B	25C	25D	25E
26	26A	26B	26C	26D	26E
27	27A	27B	27C	27D	27E
28	28A	28B	28C	28D	28E
29	29A	29B	29C	29D	29E
30	30A	30B	30C	30D	30E

Each cell has T F D options.

Time allowed — one hour.

All questions must be answered by filling in the true/false or don't know boxes on the computer marking sheet.

1 Recognised drug induced movement disorders include

A Chorea from the combined pill.
B Tremor from salbutamol (Ventolin).
C Parkinsonism from lithium.
D Acute dystonia from metoclopramide (Maxalon).
E Parkinsonian tremor from anticholinergics.

2 In pertussis

A The incubation period is less than seven days.
B Expiratory whooping is characteristic.
C Mortality is greatest in infants below six months of age.
D Antibiotics play little part in relieving symptoms.
E Immunisation is contraindicated in babies with eczema.

3 Measles vaccine

A Is quickly killed by alcohol.
B If given after the age of three years is associated with increased incidence of severe reactions.
C Should not be given to children who are allergic to eggs.
D May produce pyrexia and rash.
E Should not be given to debilitated children.

4 In anorexia nervosa

A Only females are affected.
B There is no social class difference.
C The majority are recovered within 10 years of first being diagnosed.
D There is characteristically a distorted perception of own body image.
E Depression may be a prominent feature.

5 Skin lesions which may disappear spontaneously include

A Rodent ulcer.
B Acathosis nigricans.
C Pityriasis rosea.
D Cavernous haemangioma.
E Lichen planus.

6 With simple faints is it correct to say

A Males and females are equally likely to be affected.
B A feeling of surroundings becoming dark and distant is a characteristic prodromal symptom.
C Incontinence never occurs.
D The pulse is bounding.
E Recovery occurs after a minute or two.

7 In otosclerosis

A A dominant mode of inheritance operates.
B Bilateral involvement is the rule.
C Only conductive deafness occurs.
D Stapedectomy may be indicated.
E In the majority of cases hearing aids are ineffective.

21

8 Undescended testicles

A Are as likely to undergo torsion as normally descended testicles.
B Are more common in premature than full term babies.
C If retractile will descend spontaneously when the little boy is placed in a cold bath.
D Should ideally be operated on at the age of about eight years.
E Can be successfully treated by a course of chorionic gonadotrophin (Pregnyl) injections.

9 Digoxin

A Decreases existing myocardial oxygen consumption.
B Slows the heart rate by direct action on the SA node.
C Has increased toxic effects in the presence of hypokalaemia.
D Is least effective in heart failure associated with fibrillation.
E In early overdosage can cause ectopic beats.

10 Features suggesting that an APH at 36 weeks gestation was caused by placenta praevia include

A Bright red loss.
B Associated pre-eclampsia.
C A tender uterus.
D Painless bleeding.
E A transverse lie.

11 Recognised causes of hypercalciuria include

A Osteomalacia.
B Immobilisation.
C Renal calculi.
D Sarcoidosis.
E Gout.

12 In salmonella food poisoning

A *S. agona* accounts for the majority of human infections.
B Symptoms usually develop within one to six hours of ingestion of infected food.
C Bloody diarrhoea is characteristic.
D Fatalities do not occur.
E The carrier state may be prolonged if antibiotics are given.

13 In threatened abortion

A Bleeding is as likely to occur after 12 weeks gestation as before.
B Increased parity is an aetiological factor.
C There is no increase in perinatal mortality in pregnancies which subsequently go to term.
D Strict bed rest has been proved to be effective treatment.
E Congenital malformation of the uterus is the cause in the majority of cases.

14 The following conditions are less common in breast fed infants.

A Allergic disorders.
B Dental caries.
C Cot deaths.
D Constipation.
E Gastroenteritis.

15 Phobias

A Are fears that are in voluntary control.
B Can be removed by explanation.
C Lead to avoidance of the feared situation.
D Generally respond well to desensitizing procedures.
E Are not realised by the patients to be fears that are out of proportion to the demands of the situation.

16 In acute wry neck

A The majority of cases occur in the over 40s.
B The patient characteristically wakes with his neck in a flexed rotated position.
C Radiology is diagnostic.
D There are no neurological signs.
E Manipulation has nothing to offer.

17 Depression is a recognised complication of treatment with

A Metronidazole (Flagyl)
B Corticosteroids.
C Oral contraceptives.
D Fluphenazine (Modecate).
E Appetite suppressants.

18 Characteristic features of endometriosis include

A Infertility.
B Lower social class.
C Worsening of symptoms at the menopause.
D Menorrhagia.
E A beneficial effect from combined oestrogen/progestogen therapy.

19 In the majority of cases atopic eczema

A Presents before the age of three months.
B Causes a unilateral lesion.
C Affects the popliteal and/or the antecubital fossae.
D Will clear permanently during childhood.
E Sufferers will develop asthma or hayfever in later life.

20 Recognised features of obsessional thinking include

A Persistent doubting.
B A feeling of subjective compulsion.
C Resistance to the thoughts.
D Retention of insight.
E Enjoyment by the patient.

21 In low back pain

A If more than one nerve root is involved then disc prolapse is an unlikely cause.
B Spontaneous recovery within one month is to be expected in the majority of cases.
C Caused by ankylosing spondylitis lateral flexion is typically unaffected.
D Manipulation is most effective in those with neurological involvement.
E Associated with S1 nerve root involvement the knee jerk is absent or diminished.

22 In Paget's disease of bone

A The pathological changes arise from an increase in the number and activity of osteoclasts.
B The bone pain is characteristically relieved by rest.
C Pathological fractures do not occur as bone bends rather than breaks.
D Progression to malignancy is not a risk.
E A nerve or conduction type of deafness may be produced.

23 Drugs for the prophylaxis of malaria in travellers

A Should be started at least one week prior to entering an endemic area.
B Should be taken for at least six weeks after leaving an endemic area.
C Must not be taken by pregnant women.
D Should only be taken if the traveller is going to stay in a malaria area for more than a day.
E Are guaranteed to prevent malaria.

24 Recognised side effects of chlorpromazine include

A Nasal stuffiness.
B Hyperpyrexia.
C Dystonia.
D Jaundice.
E Nausea.

25 In psittacosis

A A virus is the causative organism.
B Infection is transmitted to man from infected birds.
C A mild case may produce influenza-like symptoms.
D Clinical signs of consolidation will be found in the majority of cases.
E Tetracyclines are the treatment of choice.

26 A psychiatrist starts your patient on a monoamine oxidase inhibitor. The patient should be advised to avoid

A Chianti
B Cheddar cheese.
C Broad beans.
D Yeast extracts.
E Proprietary cough medicines.

27 With squints it is correct to say

A Children who constantly squint cannot develop true binocular vision.
B The larger the angle of squint then the more serious the effect on visual acuity.
C An inconstant squint in the early weeks of life demands immediate full investigation.
D Treatment should ideally be finished by the age of seven years.
E If a child has a squint that alternates from eye to eye then the prognosis for normal eyesight is worse than if the squint is only in one eye.

28 A Bartholin's abscess

A Is gonococcal in origin in the majority of cases.
B Is more common on the left than on the right side.
C Typically develops in the anterior part of the labium majus.
D Is most effectively treated by antibiotic therapy.
E Can be treated by marsupialisation.

29 In congenital adrenal hyperplasia

A Only females are affected.
B There is a marked fall in ACTH production.
C The enzyme most frequently affected is 21-hydroxylase.
D Virilization may occur.
E Replacement therapy similar to that required by those with primary adrenocortical insufficiency may be indicated.

30 In essential thrombocytopenia

A Adolescents and young adults are mainly affected.
B Moderate enlargement of the spleen is characteristic.
C The bleeding time is normal.
D The coagulation time is prolonged.
E Steroids are contraindicated.

THE ANSWERS TO MCQ TEST 3 BEGIN ON PAGE 40

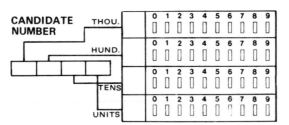

OFFICIAL USE ONLY

SURNAME	INITIALS

CANDIDATE NUMBER

THOU. 0 1 2 3 4 5 6 7 8 9
HUND. 0 1 2 3 4 5 6 7 8 9
TENS 0 1 2 3 4 5 6 7 8 9
UNITS 0 1 2 3 4 5 6 7 8 9

PAGE No.
1

T means **TRUE** F means **FALSE** D means **DO NOT KNOW**

	1A	1B	1C	1D	1E		2A	2B	2C	2D	2E
1	T F D	T F D	T F D	T F D	T F D	**2**	T F D	T F D	T F D	T F D	T F D
	3A	3B	3C	3D	3E		4A	4B	4C	4D	4E
3	T F D	T F D	T F D	T F D	T F D	**4**	T F D	T F D	T F D	T F D	T F D
	5A	5B	5C	5D	5E		6A	6B	6C	6D	6E
5	T F D	T F D	T F D	T F D	T F D	**6**	T F D	T F D	T F D	T F D	T F D
	7A	7B	7C	7D	7E		8A	8B	8C	8D	8E
7	T F D	T F D	T F D	T F D	T F D	**8**	T F D	T F D	T F D	T F D	T F D
	9A	9B	9C	9D	9E		10A	10B	10C	10D	10E
9	T F D	T F D	T F D	T F D	T F D	**10**	T F D	T F D	T F D	T F D	T F D
	11A	11B	11C	11D	11E		12A	12B	12C	12D	12E
11	T F D	T F D	T F D	T F D	T F D	**12**	T F D	T F D	T F D	T F D	T F D
	13A	13B	13C	13D	13E		14A	14B	14C	14D	14E
13	T F D	T F D	T F D	T F D	T F D	**14**	T F D	T F D	T F D	T F D	T F D
	15A	15B	15C	15D	15E		16A	16B	16C	16D	16E
15	T F D	T F D	T F D	T F D	T F D	**16**	T F D	T F D	T F D	T F D	T F D
	17A	17B	17C	17D	17E		18A	18B	18C	18D	18E
17	T F D	T F D	T F D	T F D	T F D	**18**	T F D	T F D	T F D	T F D	T F D
	19A	19B	19C	19D	19E		20A	20B	20C	20D	20E
19	T F D	T F D	T F D	T F D	T F D	**20**	T F D	T F D	T F D	T F D	T F D
	21A	21B	21C	21D	21E		22A	22B	22C	22D	22E
21	T F D	T F D	T F D	T F D	T F D	**22**	T F D	T F D	T F D	T F D	T F D
	23A	23B	23C	23D	23E		24A	24B	24C	24D	24E
23	T F D	T F D	T F D	T F D	T F D	**24**	T F D	T F D	T F D	T F D	T F D
	25A	25B	25C	25D	25E		26A	26B	26C	26D	26E
25	T F D	T F D	T F D	T F D	T F D	**26**	T F D	T F D	T F D	T F D	T F D
	27A	27B	27C	27D	27E		28A	28B	28C	28D	28E
27	T F D	T F D	T F D	T F D	T F D	**28**	T F D	T F D	T F D	T F D	T F D
	29A	29B	29C	29D	29E		30A	30B	30C	30D	30E
29	T F D	T F D	T F D	T F D	T F D	**30**	T F D	T F D	T F D	T F D	T F D

Time allowed — one hour.

All questions must be answered by filling in the true/false or don't know boxes on the computer marking sheet.

1 During lithium carbonate therapy it is correct to say

A Toxicity is unlikely to occur.
B Diuretics should be avoided.
C Blood levels should be monitored regularly.
D A goitre may develop.
E Gastrointestinal upset may be an early sign of overdosage.

2 Characteristic features of Cushing's syndrome include

A Menorrhagia.
B Hypotension.
C Skin striae.
D Muscle weakness.
E Generalised obesity.

3 Death of a patient must be reported to the coronor if the cause of death is

A Domestic accident.
B Industrial disease.
C Alcoholism.
D Suicide.
E Abortion.

4 Well recognised biochemical/haematological changes in active rheumatoid arthritis include

A Lowered serum iron.
B Abnormal electrolytes.
C Raised C reactive protein.
D Lowered serum albumin.
E Raised blood glucose.

5 An autistic child characteristically

A Dislikes a regular routine.
B Enjoys physical contact with others.
C Shows no abnormality on physical examination.
D Is echolalic.
E Lacks energy.

6 Acne

A In the majority of females is likely to flare up pre-menstrually.
B May well be worsened by exposure to sunlight.
C Is adversely affected by the eating of chocolate.
D Blackheads are inflamed lesions.
E May be treated by retinoic acid preparations.

7 In childhood orthopaedics

A When a child rises on the ball of the foot the medial longitudinal arch should become more pronounced.
B Walking with the toes turned in is a potentially serious condition requiring orthopaedic referral.
C At the age of 3 years the majority of children are mildly knock kneed.
D A normally worn shoe should have the point of maximum wear on the medial side of the heel.
E Anterior bowing of the tibia in infancy is a variation of normal.

8 In the emergency treatment of poisoning

A Saline solution is a safe first choice emetic.

B The first priority in all cases is to try to remove the poison from the stomach.

C Penicillamine is a specific antidote to iron salts.

D Petroleum products should not be removed from the stomach.

E An adult who has ingested 18 g of paracetamol can safely be managed at home.

9 Recognised metabolic changes caused by the combined pill include

A Raised serum thyroxine.

B Raised serum triglycerides.

C Vitamin B6 deficiency.

D Raised fasting blood glucose.

E Lowered plasma folate.

10 SLE (systemic lupus erythematosus)

A Onset is rare after the age of 40.

B May be exacerbated by UV light.

C May cause alopecia.

D In the majority of cases will involve the CNS.

E Should not be treated with long-term prednisolone.

11 An IUCD

A Under no circumstances should be inserted after the tenth day of the menstrual cycle.

B Insertion may be complicated by perforation of the uterus.

C Has about a 1 in 10 chance of being expelled.

D May cause increased physiological vaginal discharge.

E Fitting is not contraindicated by a past history of ectopic pregnancy.

12 It is correct to say

A Calcific deltoid bursitis gives pain equally on active and passive movements.

B Ulnar neuritis may cause thenar paralysis.

C The pain of carpal tunnel syndrome does not radiate to the elbow.

D C6 root pressure will affect the ulnar side of the arm and the little and ring fingers.

E Supraspinatus tendinitis causes pain on resisted abduction.

13 A diagnosis of conductive rather than sensorineural deafness would be supported if the deaf patient

A Spoke in a soft voice.

B Heard better if you raised your voice.

C Heard speech better in a quiet environment.

D Also complained of tinnitus.

E Heard a centrally placed (forehead) tuning fork better in his less deaf ear.

14 A three-year-old child is found on routine auscultation to have a heart murmur. Features that would suggest it was innocent include

A Diastolic in timing.

B Variation with respiration.

C Of short duration.

D Heard over a wide area of the heart.

E Associated thrill.

15 A GP should suspect alcoholism if a patient presents with

A Tongue tremor.

B Unexplained constipation.

C Noctural incontinence.

D A history of frequent job changes.

E A lowered serum gamma glutamyl transpeptidase.

16 In obesity

A Triceps skin fold thickness is a reliable estimate of degree of overweight.
B Body fat is decreased by physical training.
C Circulating levels of plasma cortisol are increased.
D Weight loss is more rapid if dietary calories are taken in frequent meals rather than just one meal per day.
E Developing in adults is due to an increase in the number of fat cells.

17 Griseofulvin

A Is effective against skin infections caused by yeasts.
B Potentiates the effects of alcohol.
C May cause headaches.
D Is less well absorbed after fatty food.
E Works best in short sharp courses.

18 Drugs which may adversely affect the fetus if given to the mother in the second or third trimester include

A Thiazide diuretics.
B Methyldopa.
C Antacids.
D Chlorpropamide.
E Soluble aspirin in high dosage.

19 In primary enuresis it is correct to say

A About 75 per cent of all children are dry by night at age three years.
B The use of antidepressants in treatment is accompanied by a high relapse rate.
C A micturating cystogram is a necessary investigation.
D Children of all social classes are affected equally.
E To avoid psychological ill effects treatment should be started as soon after age three years as possible.

20 Psychosexually it is correct to say

A Homosexuality responds well to aversion therapy in the majority of cases.
B Masturbation is a normal phase of sexual development.
C Religious orthodoxy is an important aetiological factor in the causation of impotence.
D Frigidity can only rarely be successfully treated.
E Alcohol invariably enhances sexual performance.

21 Gallstones

A Are present in about 10 to 15 per cent of the adult population of GB.
B Can be diagnosed by a history of fatty food intolerance.
C Occur with increased frequency in women taking oral contraceptives.
D Are radiopaque in the majority of cases.
E If symptomatic are best treated by cholecystectomy.

22 Characteristic features of osteomalacia include

A Tetany.
B Frontal and parietal bossing of the skull.
C Hyporeflexia.
D Muscular weakness.
E Elevated plasma phosphate levels.

23 Patients requiring treatment for the following disorders are exempt from all prescription charges

A Cardiac failure.
B Diabetes.
C Hypertension.
D Manic depressive psychosis.
E Myxoedema.

24 In a patient with prostatism the following drugs may exacerbate urinary flow problems

A Antihistamines.
B Levodopa.
C Frusemide.
D Imipramine.
E Propranolol.

25 Recognised causes of transient arthropathy include

A Rubella vaccination.
B Mumps
C Thyrotoxicosis.
D Malignancy arising in the breast.
E Dysentery.

26 In psychiatric terminology

A Verbigeration is the continuation of an activity without appropriate stimulation.
B Echopraxia means the repetition of actions seen.
C Agnosia is loss of smell caused by hysteria.
D Confabulation means the fabrication of memories.
E Hypochondria is a settled conviction of physical disease in the absence of any evidence thereof.

27 Febrile convulsions in childhood

A Will affect about 10 per cent of preschool children.
B Can be treated with rectal diazepam.
C In the majority of cases are the precursor of epilepsy.
D Are more likely to recur if the first fit is prolonged.
E Are defined as convulsions associated with a rectal temperature of 38°C or more.

28 Glaucoma

A If untreated will lead to blindness.
B Characteristically causes colourless haloes round lights.
C If mild causes the affected pupil to become smaller than its partner.
D May be aggravated by imipramine.
E Produces full cupping of the optic disc as an early feature.

29 In infertility

A The cause will be found to be in the female in about 75 per cent of cases.
B Laparoscopy is rarely of much help in eliciting causal factors.
C Clomiphene citrate may be of value where failure of ovulation is certain.
D A minimum of 40×10^6 sperms/mm^3 of semen would be considered a satisfactory number.
E If all else fails the GP can help couples arrange to adopt a child privately.

30 Myxoedema

A May lead to baldness.
B Has an association with pernicious anaemia.
C Characteristically causes a faster ankle jerk return.
D If primary gives elevated serum thyroid stimulating hormone levels.
E May cause spontaneous hypoglycaemia.

THE ANSWERS TO MCQ TEST 4 BEGIN ON PAGE 44

Answers

1 A FALSE Short duration of action and should be twice daily.

B TRUE Like all sulphonylureas mainly acts by augmenting insulin secretion.

C FALSE May give this four hours or more after feeding and usually sign of overdosage.

D TRUE As may chlorpropamide.

E FALSE Biguanides best for obese diabetics who cannot or will not lose weight

2 A FALSE Almost true but not quite.

B FALSE Urethritis precedes conjunctivitis by one to three weeks.

C TRUE Although mainly venereal in origin.

D FALSE Polyarthritis usually affecting small and medium sized joints mainly of the legs.

E FALSE Not influenced by penicillin. Tetracyclines are the drug of choice for the NSU and analgesic anti-inflammatory drugs for the arthritis.

TP Ref part A. There are very few situations in medicine where the use of the word 'always' is going to give a TRUE answer.

3 A TRUE 80 per cent plus.

B FALSE Very high.

C FALSE The fetus is capable of doing this from as early as 20 weeks of gestational life.

D FALSE Virus excreted from nasopharynx for five to seven days before and up to 10 days or more after rash.

E FALSE No viraemia so virtually no fetal risk.

4 A FALSE History of broken home or illegitimacy common.

B FALSE Not sustained but occurs in the form of episodes followed by periods of relative calmness often with considerable insight. The violence is not premeditated and is almost in the nature of a reflex.

C FALSE Hard and cold.

D TRUE 65 per cent as compared to 15 per cent of normal controls.

E FALSE See B.

TP The words common and often are used in these answers. If they and the words like them, e.g. rarely, frequently, usually, sometimes, are used in questions then the answer will nearly always be FALSE. Your knowledge, not your interpretation of the English language, is being tested.

5 A TRUE Remains rudimentary in many animals apart from in the mating season.

B TRUE Although quality of orgasm unchanged.

C TRUE It does.

D FALSE Little to distinguish carcinoma from benign hypertrophy until do PR and further investigation.

E FALSE Acid phosphatase may be elevated but even this would not be diagnostic.

6 A TRUE And reduces pepsin output.
  B FALSE With meals.
  C FALSE May well need antacids until symptoms resolve.
  D TRUE Although dosage should be reduced if there is impaired renal function.
  E TRUE Dizziness, rash and tiredness have also been reported.

7 A TRUE Degree of ST depression not related to digitalisation so cannot be used to judge dosages.
  B FALSE Reduced.
  C TRUE Sign of toxicity with every second QRS complex wide and bizarre.
  D TRUE Again a sign of toxicity.
  E TRUE A resting pulse below 65 suggests possible toxicity developing.

8 A TRUE 88 per cent are in this group.
  B FALSE The mother is, though the father usually gives tacit consent.
  C TRUE Also when a child will not go to sleep, i.e. more likely to be hit when they create problems for adults.
  D FALSE These commonly occur through children falling or knocking themselves. 73 per cent in an NSPCC survey of battered children had facial bruising.
  E TRUE They may.

9 A TRUE Generally due to failure to make the right diagnosis.
  B TRUE Nonspecific, gonococcal, post-abortal or rarely TB.
  C TRUE Also if IUCD in situ.

  D FALSE Pain is followed by bleeding.
  E FALSE Unwise as not only will cause patient discomfort but may cause rupture.

TP Where a specific figure, such as seven per cent in part A, is given then it is either the correct answer or very wide of the mark indeed. In other words if you thought the answer was from 5 to 10 per cent or so then put down true.

10 A TRUE About 45 patients per GP.
  B FALSE Baldness does not result.
  C FALSE Seronegative arthritis.
  D FALSE Too high a risk of folliculitis.
  E TRUE Then relapses after.

11 A TRUE Also sudden squints caused by mononeuropathy of ocular muscles.
  B FALSE Loss of erection may occur.
  C FALSE Diarrhoea.
  D TRUE With aching.
  E FALSE Absent or diminished.

12 A FALSE No satisfactory serum antibody test.
  B FALSE 40 times more common.
  C TRUE May be asymptomatic or give discharge with tenesmus.
  D FALSE Women often have no symptoms and when they do, examination seldom shows any abnormal features.
  E TRUE Still one of the few infections that responds well to a single dose of antibiotics.

13 A TRUE It is.
  B FALSE Sterile fluid.
  C FALSE In two-thirds of cases the adenoids are either small or have been removed.

D TRUE   Easy. Better results than myringotomy provided the grommet remains in situ.

E FALSE   Gives conductive loss only.

14 A TRUE   Also vocalises and turns head to sound.

B TRUE   Also able to lie prone with weight on forearms.

C TRUE   Also can attract attention by coughing and turn head to sound below level of ears.

D FALSE   Not until about 10 months for this.

E FALSE   Four to five clear words at this time but no sentence until 21 to 24 months.

15 A TRUE   May well blame someone for the death.

B TRUE   Sevenfold in first year after the death (Rees and Lutkins survey).

C TRUE   Also of panic and unreality.

D TRUE   Also may complain of some of the deceased's symptoms.

E FALSE   Readjustment within about six months.

16 A FALSE   Pattern is for loss of voluntary and involuntary movement.

B FALSE   Remain flexor.

C FALSE   Plastic or cogwheel rigidity.

D FALSE   Most prominent at rest but subsides during sleep.

E TRUE   Anticholinergic drugs help to reduce both this and tremor.

17 A FALSE   Less than 0.5 per cent of the body K^+ is in the plasma.

B FALSE   Loop diuretics produce a smaller fall than thiazides (for equivalent diuresis).

C TRUE   Increased intake balanced by increased urinary excretion.

D FALSE   Reduces it both by renal action and by reducing dose of diuretic required.

E TRUE   Serum K^+ should be corrected if falls below 3 mmol/litre and K^+ sparing diuretics are more effective than K^+ supplements.

18 A FALSE   The patient will prefer to sit upright.

B TRUE   And arrhythmias especially if injected too fast.

C FALSE   Up to 40 per cent without risk and 100 per cent if no lung disease present.

D TRUE   Removes fluid from the lungs by producing dilation of systemic veins.

E TRUE   Dangerous as raises BP.

TP No one should get part A wrong unless they have not read the question carefully. There are no trick questions and the obvious meaning of a statement is the correct one.

19 A FALSE   Winter though other causes of infantile gastroenteritis manifest in late summer.

B FALSE   High temperature common.

C FALSE   This would suggest salmonella. Watery with rotavirus.

D FALSE   Dioralyte/diluted Coco cola/ sweetened water but all with no salt or enough for a dilute solution approximating to half normal saline.

E FALSE   Ineffective and produce high incidence of side-effects.

TP Although all five answers here are FALSE it is, in fact, quite difficult technically to produce five equally plausible FALSE statements about one topic. There are unlikely to be more than two or three questions in the paper with all FALSE answers.

20 A FALSE If anything the reverse is the case though most patients present with both.

B FALSE Weakened and wasted.

C TRUE So adduction of the thumb can only be achieved through flexor pollicis longus causing flexion of the thumb tip (Froments' sign).

D TRUE With impaired sensation over little finger and ulnar side of ring finger.

E TRUE As opposed to thenar involvement in carpal tunnel syndrome.

21 A FALSE Schizophrenic feature.

B FALSE Quite the reverse as tend to feel hopeless and unworthy.

C FALSE May help at first but later is quite ineffective.

D TRUE Many patients describe the slowness of passage of time.

E FALSE No alteration in duration though content becomes gloomy or frightening.

22 A FALSE Incidence of this increased in pill users but only a relative contraindication.

B FALSE Although LFT's before and after commencing the pill would be wise.

C FALSE Decreases incidence of this.

D FALSE Though thalassaemia itself or sickle cell anaemia are probably contraindications.

E TRUE It is.

23 A FALSE Natural and synthetic narcotics, amphetamines and other stimulants are controlled.

B FALSE Both words and figures.

C TRUE According to a previous High Court Judgement.

D TRUE Must inform chief MO of the Drug Branch.

E TRUE It has.

24 A FALSE Was one per cent at 10 years in 1939. Now 60 per cent at 20 years.

B FALSE In contrast to patients with coeliac disease appetite is often increased and may be voracious.

C TRUE Well known.

D FALSE Lower particularly if associated steatorrhoea or failure to thrive.

E FALSE About 10 per cent develop mild diabetes.

25 A FALSE Dilation with possible rise in intraocular pressure.

B FALSE Reduced vagal tone so increased heart rate.

C TRUE All secretions except milk are diminished.

D TRUE And possible retention.

E FALSE Smooth muscle is relaxed.

26 A FALSE Very pale because no urobilinogen in them.

B FALSE None is being formed.

C FALSE Generally markedly raised.

D FALSE Often raised in obstructive jaundice and certainly not lowered.

E FALSE Marked pruritis caused by accumulation of bile salts in the blood.

TP All the answers to this question happen to be FALSE. Remember they could equally well all be TRUE or in any combination of TRUE or FALSE.

27 A FALSE Great restlessness, sleeplessness and fear.
   B TRUE With tachycardia and slight pyrexia.
   C FALSE Persistent craving throughout.
   D TRUE Often widely so.
   E FALSE Coarse generalised tremor.

28 A TRUE Because the expansion of the plasma volume is proportionately greater than any rise in the red cell mass.
   B FALSE Human chorionic gonadotrophin does.
   C FALSE Stomach emptying time is almost doubled.
   D FALSE It does not. The fetus is a perfect parasite.
   E FALSE They are the same.

29 A FALSE Circumcorneal.
   B FALSE Contraction from reflex spasm of the sphincter.
   C FALSE Light seems positively hurtful to the eye.

D TRUE Adhesions between iris and the anterior lens surface.
E TRUE Clumps of pus cells in the anterior chamber.

30 A TRUE First and second sounds clearly distinct from the murmur.
   B FALSE Pansystolic running into first and second sounds.
   C TRUE Similar to that of aortic stenosis but extends through aortic second sound.
   D FALSE Pansystolic heard best at lower left sternal edge.
   E FALSE Harsh pansystolic often with a thrill.

TP The answers to this type of question can be worked out though generally only with the expenditure of a fair amount of time. Before the exam you must decide whether to do each question as you come to it or whether you will leave potentially time-consuming questions until the end of the paper. The advantage of the latter course of action is that you will not miss easy marks by running out of time before you have attempted all the questions.

MCQ
TEST 2

Answers

1 A TRUE One reason for using with caution in young females.
  B FALSE Interferes with folate metabolism.
  C TRUE Common.
  D TRUE With ataxia is cardinal initial symptom of overdosage.
  E FALSE This can occur with sulthiame.

2 A FALSE Generally gradual in previously active old ladies.
  B TRUE With painful restriction of shoulder movement.
  C FALSE Muscle pain but no arthritis.
  D FALSE Usually absent and no objective evidence of muscle weakness.
  E FALSE Good response.

3 A TRUE Over 90 per cent of women in the 21 to 34 age group for example.

B FALSE Declines.

C FALSE Not so, though it is the more intelligent ones that consult a doctor.

D FALSE No evidence for this at all.

E FALSE May be increased in those with diastolic greater than 130 mm Hg.

4 A TRUE Frequently observed but also risk of paranoia or severe depression.

B TRUE Affects about one-third of patients.

C FALSE Not so.

D FALSE This area is responsible for the interpretation and correlation of sensation.

E TRUE May feel euphoric or elated.

5 A TRUE Follicles seem to be switched off but even after many years can start to produce hair again.

B TRUE Definite association with immune system disorders especially thyroid disease.

C TRUE Also in Down's syndrome and those with vitiligo.

D FALSE Often induces atrophy of the scalp.

E FALSE Within six months.

6 A FALSE Characteristic of only some fevers. Usually the skin is hot and dry though sweating may occur when the temperature falls.

B TRUE Error of only up to 0.1°C though I doubt if any doctor waits that long!

C TRUE It is.

D TRUE Though if prolonged may cause permanent brain damage.

E FALSE Defined as greater than 37.2°C.

7 A TRUE If any nappy rash fails to respond to simple measures, then assume *Candida* infection present.

B TRUE Because not in contact with urine or stool.

C FALSE Raise temperature of the nappy area and so promote microbial growth.

D FALSE Staphyloccal infection. Small red perianal satellite lesions indicate monilia.

E TRUE Soothing, protective and astringent.

8 A TRUE Active against a wide variety of protozoa and many obligate anaerobic bacteria.

B FALSE With or shortly after to decrease GI upsets.

C TRUE Effect caused by some of its metabolites.

D TRUE Almost all cases respond to single dose or 200 mg TID for one week.

E TRUE May have a disulfiram-like effect during therapy.

9 A FALSE Common but under-diagnosed condition affecting 33 to 40 per cent of women.

B FALSE Will after oophorectomy.

C FALSE This is the normal situation. In PMT a relative deficiency of progesterone (as compared to oestrogen) is a possible cause.

D FALSE Helps fluid retention symptoms but no effect on depression, irritability and so on.

E TRUE Most characteristic feature is recurrence of symptoms at regular intervals of about one month with relief with onset of menstruation.

10 A TRUE Although may also occur at rest.

B FALSE Generally not for more than 15 minutes. If prolonged think of RA.

C FALSE Suggests acute gout or sepsis.

D TRUE Almost always present and genu valgum or varum may result from severe disease.

E FALSE Limp only when disease is advanced.

11 A TRUE Also occipital headaches.

B FALSE Feature of carotid insufficiency.

C TRUE Caused by generalised loss of muscle tone.

D FALSE No connection.

E TRUE Well known.

12 A TRUE Relative risk of 2.5 over non-users. Similar risk in pill users.

B FALSE Neither protects nor causes.

C FALSE Will delay accelerated bone loss in postmenopausal osteoporotic women for a limited time.

D TRUE Many studies suggest this.

E FALSE Helps alleviate symptoms due to this.

13 A FALSE 10 to 1 male predominance.

B TRUE Anyone with this requires expert examination, regardless of their age.

C TRUE Main aetiological factor.

D TRUE 5 year survival of 70 per cent after irradiation alone.

E FALSE Always not sometimes and may be a bar to complete social rehabilitation.

14 A TRUE From metabolic acidosis.

B FALSE Loss of tissue turgor becomes apparent when a child is about 2.5 to 5 per cent dehydrated.

C TRUE With baby in nappies may well be apparent to mum.

D TRUE If recent weight recording available then accurate objective assessment can be made.

E FALSE Sunken with sunken eyes.

15 A FALSE The mental symptoms generally occur in a setting of clear consciousness.

B TRUE Impaired with decreased ability to learn new material.

C TRUE Recent more than remote.

D TRUE 'Emotional incontinence'.

E TRUE Ultimately affects all spheres.

16 A TRUE You have problems if you don't know this.

B TRUE Also fasting greater than 120 mg/dl (6.7 mmol/l).

C FALSE 8 units. Would be 16 if 4 marks of 80 strength.

D FALSE Is in juvenile onset where disease present for many years.

E FALSE Soft exudates, fine new vessels, fibrous patches and rubeosis of the iris signify this.

17 A TRUE Increased sedation plus risk of paralytic ileus especially in the elderly.

B FALSE May actually increase antidepressant effect.

C TRUE Loss of antihypertensive activity.

D TRUE Metabolism inhibited and phenytoin toxicity may occur.

E TRUE Serious risk of cardiac dysrhythmia.

18 A TRUE Especially uniovular twins.

B FALSE Commoner in multips.

C TRUE Anencephaly and spina bifida predominantly.

D TRUE Distinct possibility though not as great as in the case of twins.

E TRUE Occurs with anything which prevents the presenting part fitting closely into the lower segment.

19 A TRUE And brain damage.

B FALSE As good an antipyretic as aspirin.

C FALSE Increased insensible loss occurring.

D FALSE Should use warm water as colder water causes peripheral vasoconstriction and shivering and so may increase temperature even further.

E TRUE May well need i.v. fluids and alpha blocking drugs.

20 A TRUE Also other life stresses, e.g. bereavement, separation, loss of job.

B TRUE Also depression, alcoholism, organic brain syndrome.

C FALSE Attempts are most often made by young females but it is the depressive over 40 who is most likely to succeed.

D FALSE Ideas of guilt and unworthiness.

E TRUE Also unemployment and social isolation.

21 A TRUE This would be likely in peripheral vascular disease.

B TRUE See A.

C FALSE Pallor with elevation of the foot is what is expected.

D FALSE This would occur with DVT.

E FALSE Not related to the presence of intermittent claudication.

22 A TRUE Most cervical flexion and extension takes place at C5-6 and C6-7 intervertebral discs so bulk degenerative changes found here.

B FALSE Motor involvement gives weakness, wasting and fasciculation.

C TRUE If first thoracic root involved.

D TRUE From spinal cord involvement.

E FALSE Usually helps but likelihood of relapse when the collar is discarded.

23 A TRUE After measles is the commonest disease notified.

B FALSE Not so.

C TRUE Also acute meningitis.

D TRUE 9000 cases with 3 deaths in England and Wales in 1976.

E FALSE Not so.

24 A TRUE It is.

B TRUE The same process involving the distal epiphysis of the second metatarsal bone is Freiburg's disease and the navicular is Kohler's disease.

C FALSE Child complains of painful hip.

D TRUE Correct statement.

E TRUE Usually noticed first by the parents.

25 A FALSE Contraindicated. Best for chronic plaques.

B FALSE Dose related irritancy varying from mild erythema to blistering.

C TRUE This is a zinc compound paste often used with coal tar or dithranol.

D TRUE And normal skin purplish-brown.

E FALSE Start low (0.1 per cent) and work up to 0.5 per cent if no adverse effects.

26 A FALSE This is the laboured breathing of ketoacidosis. Normal breathing in hypoglycaemia.

B FALSE Ketoacidosis would give this.
C TRUE Characteristic feature.
D TRUE And rapid.
E FALSE This and vomiting are often associated with ketoacidosis.

27 A TRUE For clinical and medico-legal reasons.

B TRUE They do. Local anaesthetics, which also relieve pain, should generally not be used more than once as they may delay healing and promote further damage.

C TRUE Many chemical burns have late complications because of retained particles.

D FALSE Less examination the better as attempts to determine the extent of the wound may increase the damage.

E TRUE If pupil is deformed assume penetration. Unfortunately a round pupil does not rule it out.

28 A FALSE Is an extension of the endo-cervical columnar epithelium into the vagina.

B FALSE Commonly and normally develop during pregnancy.

C FALSE Present in at least one third of baby girls probably from exposure to maternal oestrogen in utero.

D TRUE Essentially increased normal secretion.

E FALSE It does not.

29 A FALSE Memory unimpaired though lack of attention may make it appear faulty.

B TRUE Helpful diagnostic feature.
C FALSE May occur but by no means characteristic.
D FALSE Little or no insight.
E FALSE Depressive rather than schizophrenic feature.

30 A FALSE Usually 140 to 180 but may range from 100 to 220.

B TRUE 1:1 AV conduction or 2:1 AV block in the higher rate range.

C TRUE Production of copious volumes of pale urine.

D TRUE Carotid sinus pressure/pharyngeal irritation attempted with the patient in bed.

E FALSE Still preferred to verapamil by many cardiologists for restoration of sinus rhythm.

Answers

1 A TRUE   Also from anticonvulsant therapy.

  B TRUE   Common dose related adverse effect of drugs that stimulate beta adrenoceptors.

  C TRUE   Responds to reduction of dosage.

  D TRUE   Should not be given to children as they are unduly susceptible to this.

  E FALSE   These enhance dopamine activity and so will help reduce tremor.

2 A FALSE   About 10 to 14.

  B FALSE   Inspiratory.

  C TRUE   11 deaths in 1978 epidemic.

  D TRUE   Although they do appear to shorten the period of infectivity.

  E FALSE   It is not.

3 A TRUE   Also ether and detergents so wash site with water only.

  B FALSE   Risk lessened.

  C TRUE   Attenuated virus cultured on egg protein.

  D TRUE   Usually on eighth day in about 5 to 10 per cent of children.

  E FALSE   Especially valuable but modified by simultaneous passive immunisation.

4 A FALSE   One in 15 or so are male.

  B FALSE   Much more likely in higher social classes but if does occur in IV or V then poorer prognosis.

  C TRUE   50 to 60 per cent with 2 to

5 per cent death rate (suicide, inanition) and rest still chronically ill.

  D TRUE   Gross overestimation.

  E TRUE   With feelings of guilt, isolation and suicidal thoughts.

5 A FALSE   Nonsense.

  B FALSE   This is a recognised skin manifestation of visceral carcinoma.

  C TRUE   After about three months.

  D TRUE   90 per cent resolve by the age of eight years, unlike capillary haemangioma which do not resolve.

  E TRUE   On average persist for about six months though in 10 per cent persist for years.

6 A FALSE   More commonly females.

  B TRUE   It is.

  C FALSE   May occur if bladder full, though not as commonly as in epilepsy.

  D FALSE   Small volume pulse.

  E TRUE   Attack short with rapid recovery and no sequelae.

7 A TRUE   Although with incomplete penetrance.

  B TRUE   As is the progressive course.

  C FALSE   Get sensorineural deafness if the otosclerotic process involves the bone around the cochlea.

  D TRUE   90 per cent chance of regaining almost normal hearing after this operation.

  E FALSE   Generally very effective.

8 A FALSE More likely especially in the inguinal extopic position.

B TRUE 10 per cent at birth, 2 per cent at puberty and 0.2 per cent in adults.

C FALSE Really? A hot bath is more appropriate.

D FALSE Ideally five though there is evidence two may be best for future unimpaired fertility.

E FALSE Treatment surgical. It is doubtful if hormones can have any effect on testicles which have not descended because of mechanical problems.

9 A FALSE Increases force of contraction of ventricular muscle without a corresponding increase in oxygen consumption but there is no decrease.

B TRUE And vagal action when heart in sinus rhythm.

C TRUE Elderly people and those on diuretic therapy are especially at risk.

D FALSE Is particularly effective in this situation.

E TRUE Often with vomiting and slowing of the pulse.

10 A TRUE Always bright and only darkens after the episode of bleeding has finished.

B FALSE No connection.

C FALSE Soft, non-contracting and non-tender unlike the hard and tender uterus in accidental haemorrhage.

D TRUE A characteristic feature.

E TRUE High presenting part with oblique or transverse lie commonly associated.

11 A FALSE Vitamin D overdose or sensitivity.

B TRUE Maintain high fluid intake and avoid excess calcium intake if prolonged immobilization likely.

C FALSE Effect not cause.

D TRUE Also neoplasia, myelomatosis.

E FALSE Gives hyperuricaemia.

12 A FALSE *S. typhimurium* is the commonest agent.

B FALSE Rapid onset would be typical of staphylococcal food poisoning. With salmonellae symptoms begin within 48 hours.

C FALSE No blood.

D FALSE 45 deaths in 1975 mainly in children and the elderly.

E TRUE Also these organisms develop multiple drug resistance.

13 A FALSE 80 per cent before 12 weeks.

B TRUE As is increased age.

C FALSE Three times higher than in women with no bleeding.

D FALSE It may be usual to keep the patient in bed while red loss persists but there is no good evidence that it does any good.

E FALSE Chromosomal abnormality of the fetus is.

14 A TRUE Especially eczema and asthma.

B TRUE They are.

C TRUE 3,000 pa in Great Britain but very few are breast fed.

D TRUE Also, bottle fed babies may develop obstruction due to milk plugs.

E TRUE Stools contain acetate buffer and so present a hostile environment to gram negative organisms.

15 A FALSE Irrational fears beyond any voluntary control.

B FALSE Neither explanation nor reason will remove these fears.

C TRUE Strong tendency for subjects to do this.

D TRUE Especially animal and specific situational phobias.

E FALSE Good insight retained.

16 A FALSE Usually in young adults.

B TRUE Often with mid or upper cervical tenderness.

C FALSE Shows loss of normal cervical lordosis but nothing else.

D TRUE Correct statement.

E FALSE Frequently lessens time needed for improvement.

17 A TRUE Also griseofulvin and sulphonamides though mechanism unclear.

B TRUE With suicide risk.

C TRUE Possibly enhances tryptophan breakdown or pyridoxine deficiency.

D TRUE Many reports of schizophrenics becoming severely depressed and committing suicide after depot injections. Mood change appears immediately and is of variable duration.

E TRUE Like benzodiazepines, opiates and alcohol, depression generally occurs during attempted withdrawal of the drug.

18 A TRUE 50 to 70 per cent of affected women are childless but difficult to say which is cause and which effect.

B FALSE Described as a disease of the rich.

C FALSE Almost always becomes quiescent then.

D TRUE Excessive bleeding in the large majority of cases.

E TRUE Large doses given continuously suppress ovulation and menstruation and often give good results.

19 A FALSE Generally in the first or second years of life and unusual before three months.

B FALSE Symmetrical eruption.

C TRUE Face, neck, wrists and hands also commonly involved.

D TRUE In up to 95 per cent of cases.

E FALSE Up to 10 per cent of children have eczema but only a small number will develop asthma or hayfever.

20 A TRUE This can occur in normal people if physically ill or very tired.

B TRUE ⎫
C TRUE ⎬ These are the three essential elements in the medical definition of an obsession.
D TRUE ⎭

E FALSE Disturbing and often very distressing.

21 A TRUE Only rarely will a single prolapse compress more than one root.

B TRUE 90 per cent in one survey.

C FALSE This is limited early in the disease unlike disc lesions and degenerative disease.

D FALSE Contraindicated in these cases and those with any spinal instability.

E FALSE Affects ankle jerk. L3–4 lesions for knee jerk.

22 A TRUE   Increased bone resorption so get compensatory increase in bone formation with bone enlarged and soft.

B FALSE   So it can keep the patient awake at night.

C FALSE   The abnormal bone is often the site for spontaneous fractures.

D FALSE   Almost all cases of osteogenic sarcoma in adults arise from Paget's although it is an uncommon complication.

E TRUE   Frequently.

23 A FALSE   Start from day before entry.

B TRUE   Needed for this long as incubation period is 6 to 42 days.

C FALSE   Parasite can cross placental barrier. Proguanil safe.

D FALSE   One bite by one mosquito is all that is needed.

E FALSE   They are not. Consider diagnosis in any febrile returned traveller.

24 A TRUE   Also dry mouth and other atropine-like effects.

B FALSE   May impair thermoregulation in the elderly leading to hypothermia.

C TRUE   Extrapyramidal syndromes are probably the most important side-effect.

D TRUE   A reversible sensitivity reaction.

E FALSE   Is an anti-emetic.

25 A FALSE   A bacterium *Chlamydia psittaci.*

B TRUE   Especially parrots and parakeets.

C TRUE   Probably the rule although diagnosis often will not be made.

D FALSE   Physical signs of pneumonia tend to be sparse and may well only be localized fine creps.

E TRUE   Early treatment may be life saving.

26 A TRUE   These amine containing foods may cause hypertensive crisis within one to two hours of ingestion. Severe headache, nausea, sweating and flushing occur.
  B TRUE
  C TRUE
  D TRUE

E TRUE   Ephedrine and similar agents found in cough medicines and nasal decongestant drops are dangerous.

27 A TRUE   Although of less importance than one might think because of infant's ability to adapt.

B FALSE   A small angle squint may well have as severe visual effects as one that is severe cosmetically. Underlines the need to look actively for squints.

C FALSE   Until a baby has learnt to look at objects inconstant squints are common.

D TRUE   After this really only gets cosmetic improvement.

E FALSE   If constant squint in one eye then image disregarded and only one eye will see normally. If alternating squint then each eye will only have temporary problems and vision will be normal.

28 A FALSE   Normal bowel flora most often involved.

B TRUE   For some unknown reason.

C FALSE   Distends the posterior and middle parts.

D FALSE   Once abscess formed little

43

place for antibiotics and surgery indicated.

E TRUE Operation of choice giving
immediate relief of pain and
resolution of infection within
a few days.

29 A FALSE Though mildly affected males
may not be detected at birth.
B FALSE Reduced circulating cortisol
levels stimulate ACTH production.
C TRUE Required for biosynthesis of
both cortisol and aldosterone
but not androgen.
D TRUE Because of increased androgen production.

E TRUE Need sufficient glucocorti-
coid to turn off ACTH and
cut androgen production.
May well also need fludro-
cortisone.

30 A TRUE Particularly girls.
B FALSE In about one third of cases
it becomes just palpable.
C FALSE Is prolonged.
D FALSE Clot retraction is poor but
coagulation time is normal.
E FALSE Should be tried first though
if complete remission does
not occur then splenectomy
probably indicated.

MCQ
TEST 4

Answers

1 A FALSE Occurs readily.
B TRUE As toxicity is worsened by
salt depletion (treated by
stopping drug and giving salt
plus fluids).
C TRUE Especially in the early stages
and aim for 0.6 to 1 mmol/l.
D TRUE Also hypothyroidism.
E TRUE Anorexia, nausea, abdominal
pain, V and D.

2 A FALSE Complete amenorrhoea.
B FALSE Hypertension and oedema
are frequent.
C TRUE Wide purple striae over abdo-

men and flanks.
D TRUE Generally marked.
E FALSE Fat trunk but slender limbs.

3 A TRUE Also after industrial accidents
or RTAs.
B TRUE Or if a patient suffered from
a pensioned disability.
C TRUE Or if due to drugs or poisons.
D TRUE Also if there is any accusa-
tion of negligence against a
doctor.
E TRUE Although the Abortion Act
allows it in certain circum-

stances abortion is still against the law.

4 A TRUE   Nearly always low as a result of inflammatory activity.
   B FALSE   Normal though in severe cases blood urea is raised.
   C TRUE   More sensitive measure than the ESR.
   D TRUE   A rising albumin is as useful as a falling ESR as a guide to progress.
   E FALSE   Unaffected.

5 A FALSE   Very upset if routine broken.
   B FALSE   Solitary.
   C TRUE   Although examination may be difficult as child becomes possessive of the examining instruments.
   D TRUE   Tendency to repeat the last thing that has been heard.
   E FALSE   Excessive energy and appears to need little sleep.

6 A TRUE   About two thirds notice a flare-up of spots one to seven days premenstrually.
   B FALSE   Sunlight has a favourable influence.
   C FALSE   No real evidence of this.
   D FALSE   Whiteheads are the forerunners of the papulo/pustular element.
   E TRUE   Act to produce a more primitive form of keratin which is more loosely bound to its neighbours and separates easily after two to three weeks of treatment reducing the number of whiteheads.

7 A TRUE   Flat foot which is in the normal physiological range should disappear.

   B FALSE   By the age of six years intoeing will correct itself in all but a very few children.
   C TRUE   75 per cent have more than 2.5 cm of knock knee and in over 20 per cent it is more than 5 mm. (Distance between the medial malleoli with the knees extended.)
   D FALSE   At the back of the heel to the outer side of the midline. Moderately severe knock knees would wear out the inner side of the shoe.
   E FALSE   Rare and indicates some serious condition requiring urgent radiology and orthopaedic advice.

8 A FALSE   Increasing evidence that it is dangerous because of possible death from hypernatraemia.
   B FALSE   First priority must always be respiratory function.
   C FALSE   Desferrioxamine is.
   D TRUE   More dangerous in the lungs than in the stomach so best left alone.
   E FALSE   Serious delayed action effects (liver damage) are to be expected and patient should be in hospital.

9 A TRUE   Laboratory needs to know if a woman is on the pill to prevent misdiagnosis.
   B TRUE   Long term effect on atheroma unknown but may predispose to CVA.
   C TRUE   Possible mechanism for depression and loss of libido.
   D FALSE   Lowers fasting glucose though may elevate postprandial levels.

45

E TRUE   May very rarely get megalo-blastic anaemia caused by the pill.

10 A TRUE   And 9 to 1 females to males.
   B TRUE   Commoner in Negro races and sunny climes.
   C TRUE   Commoner than the butter-fly rash.
   D TRUE   In up to two-thirds of patients with mainly neuropsychiatric disturbances.
   E FALSE   Most patients require small maintenance doses and high doses when disease active.

11 A FALSE   Usual to insert before this time but many factors may point to immediate insertion.
   B TRUE   Most perforations occur at this time.
   C TRUE   Risk highest in first year; de-clines markedly with increas-ing age and parity.
   D TRUE   It may.
   E FALSE   It most certainly is.

12 A FALSE   Almost full passive move-ment possible but severe pain on active abduction.
   B FALSE   Hypothenar.
   C FALSE   May radiate up even to the shoulder.
   D FALSE   This is C8. C6 is radial/thumb and index.
   E TRUE   And painful arc on active abduction.

13 A TRUE   In conductive deafness voice sounds loud to its owner who thus tends to speak quietly.
   B TRUE   Will help if conductive but no difference if sensorineural.
   C FALSE   With conductive speech often hears better in noisy environ-ment because speaker raises his voice.
   D FALSE   No diagnostic significance.
   E FALSE   Probably sensorineural. If heard tuning fork better in his deafer ear then conduc-tive.

14 A FALSE   All these require further in-vestigation.
   B TRUE   Also with posture.
   C TRUE   Usually midsystole and ejec-tion in type.
   D FALSE   Generally over a limited area and not well conducted.
   E FALSE   Rest of cardiac examina-tion should be negative.

15 A TRUE   Also the shakes and sweats.
   B FALSE   Unexplained diarrhoea.
   C TRUE   Also nocturia.
   D TRUE   Also driving offences, finan-cial worries.
   E FALSE   Elevated if disturbed liver metabolism due to alcohol abuse.

16 A TRUE   Although multiple skin folds are even more reliable.
   B TRUE   Fat decreased but lean tissue mass increased so weight may not change.
   C FALSE   Unchanged.
   D FALSE   Rate of loss unaffected but glucose tolerance and blood cholesterol levels are signifi-cantly improved by eating three to six times per day rather than once.
   E FALSE   In adults get increase in existing fat cell size while in children get increased num-ber of cells.

17 A FALSE   Inactive against yeasts.

B TRUE   Also diminishes the effects of anticoagulants.

C TRUE   Common side-effect decreased by taking the main dose at bedtime.

D FALSE   Aids absorption.

E FALSE   Needs six weeks for skin infections and up to one year for nail infections.

18 A TRUE   Thrombocytopenic purpura may develop.

B FALSE   Safer than diuretics and probably safer than betablockers.

C FALSE   No evidence of this.

D TRUE   All sulphonylureas carry the risk of neonatal hypoglycaemia. Tolbutamide is safer than most because of its short half-life.

E TRUE   Risk of bleeding due to platelet dysfunction and depression of factor 12.

19 A TRUE   50 per cent or so at two and 90 per cent by five.

B TRUE   Suppresses wetting completely in about 30 per cent of cases and many of these will be wet again three months after stopping therapy.

C FALSE   This is delayed normal development and less than 3 per cent will have organic disease.

D FALSE   Commonest in IV and V.

E FALSE   See A and C. Treatment is indicated only in older children.

20 A FALSE   Was in vogue a few years ago but results largely disappointing.

B TRUE   It is.

C TRUE   Especially primary but also main factor in about 15 per cent of secondary impotent men.

D FALSE   Treatment successful in about half of cases.

E FALSE   May allay inhibitions in some but in general impairs both erection and ejaculation.

21 A TRUE   Females two to three times more than males.

B FALSE   Occurs as frequently in patients without gallstones.

C TRUE   And those on HRT.

D FALSE   10 to 30 per cent are by virtue of their calcium content.

E TRUE   Easy.

22 A FALSE   Occasionally the plasma Ca^{++} level is low enough to produce this but it is by no means characteristic.

B FALSE   This occurs in rickets.

C TRUE   Well known.

D TRUE   Follows fatigue and stiffness.

E FALSE   Generally lowered.

23 A FALSE   Nor for chronic respiratory diseases.

B TRUE   Official reasoning is that exempt conditions are those that require replacement of a chemical.

C FALSE   Not so.

D FALSE   Epilepsy is the only neuro-psychiatric disorder exempted though the reason why is not at all clear.

E TRUE   Though not thyrotoxicosis (see answer B).

24 A TRUE   Most antihistamines have some anticholinergic effects especially promethazine,

pheniramine and diphenhydramine.

B FALSE   Anticholinergic parkinsonian drugs do.

C TRUE   Sudden diuresis in these patients may provoke retention.

D TRUE   Tricyclics are strong anticholinergics. Tetracyclics to be preferred in this situation.

E FALSE   No effect in this area.

25 A TRUE   As many as 40 per cent of adult females may develop this in second or third week post vaccination.

B TRUE   Especially in an overt attack in boys.

C FALSE   Although rarely may occur at the onset of mvxoedema.

D TRUE   Any type though especially bronchus, prostate and breast.

E TRUE   Can develop after the diarrhoea has settled.

26 A FALSE   Is a flow of unconnected words.

B TRUE   One aspect of automatic obedience.

C FALSE   Means failure to recognise.

D TRUE   It does.

E TRUE   Easy. Most common in depression but also in schizophrenia, hysteria or chronic anxiety state.

27 A FALSE   About 3 per cent.

B TRUE   If i.v. not possible then rectal quicker than i.m. Use i.v. preparation in syringe without needle and can be used by parents in recurrent cases.

C FALSE   About 1 in 6 will go on to have afebrile attacks

D TRUE   Or if family history of epilepsy or febrile fits.

E TRUE   Correct statement.

28 A TRUE   Early diagnosis and treatment are therefore crucial.

B FALSE   Invariably coloured or 'rainbows'.

C FALSE   Larger than its partner.

D TRUE   There are 50 or more drugs in common use which can cause or aggravate glaucoma.

E FALSE   By the time this appears the disease is far advanced.

29 A FALSE   About one-third the male, one-third the female and rest a combination of both.

B FALSE   50 per cent plus of patients will be found to have clinical unsuspected pathology.

C TRUE   Will reverse this in about one-third of cases (so long as failure of ovulation is not due to an early menopause).

D TRUE   Though volume, motility and number of abnormal forms all have to be considered as well.

E FALSE   1975 Childrens' Act made privately arranged adoptions illegal.

30 A TRUE   Hair lifeless, coarse and sparse and falls progressively.

B TRUE   10 per cent of patients with spontaneous myxoedema have PA.

C FALSE   Sluggish and reduced with delayed return.

D TRUE   Feedback mechanism to pituitary not operating.

E TRUE   Possibly from failure of mobilisation of glucose from liver glycogen.

Modified Essay Question or MEQ

The MEQ is an original development by the examiners of the RCGP of the patient-management problem type of examination format widely used in North America and Australasia. The papers are normally based on a real case and the format is the familiar one in which an evolving clinical problem is unfolded stage by stage. The participant is expected to respond in the appropriate manner by eliciting further information via history or physical examination; speculate on the diagnostic possibilities; order relevant investigations; come to a working diagnosis; advise and counsel the patient and his family; intervene appropriately by mobilising relations, nursing or social services; refer to specialists or prescribe drugs or aids; and show an awareness of risk factors in a situation by demonstrating an ability to anticipate problems which might be expected to arise in the future.

The MEQ has been demonstrated to be an excellent tool for exploring the mixture of clinical, behavioural and management skills which together make up the art of general practice. The format is also very suitable for use as an educational aid for small groups of trainees or experienced general practitioners.

In this chapter you are provided with four complete examination-style MEQs, each of which should take one hour and fifteen minutes to complete. You should try to work under examination conditions, allowing the appropriate time, and not aiming to complete more than one MEQ at a sitting. Unless the question specifically states that the answer must be written in prose, e.g. a letter to a consultant, the MEQ is best answered as a series of headings and points since this enables the examiners to mark more easily by applying the marking schedules, and takes you less time to write.

After the four MEQs in this book the papers are repeated, this time with suggested marking schedules and weighting of questions in the total paper. You may well differ in the weighting which you would yourself apply to the relative parts of the paper but we have endeavoured to give some indication of the likely distribution of marks in the MRCGP exam. Remember that pure factual knowledge is tested particularly in the MCQ and therefore extra stress is placed in marking the MEQ on those facets of management which cannot be examined in any other type of written paper. Similarly, you may wish to repudiate some of our suggested answers but remember that we have carefully checked our references and, in order to prove us wrong, you should check your own references and not accept your own fallible opinion. Try to be honest when marking your own paper or, even better, ask one or two colleagues to do the marking for you. Points about technique of answering questions and the way to approach the different types of question are noted on each page together with the marking schedules.

It is difficult to be precise about pass marks but as a general indication you should assume that 55 per cent or more represents a comfortable pass whilst 40 per cent or less spells probable failure. Attention to approach and technique may maximise the score but is no substitute for wide clinical experience and competence in general practice.

Instructions

1 There are 10 questions in this and in the subsequent three papers.

2 Answers should be brief, legible and concise. Total time allowed is **one hour and fifteen minutes** per Test.

3 Answers should be written in the space provided.

4 In those questions where a definite number of answers are asked for do not give more answers than are requested.

5 You are warned not to alter your answers after completing the whole MEQ and not to look through the paper before you start. This may distort your natural assessment of the case and cause you to lose marks.

6 The MEQ is a test of your practical approach to a developing general practice problem and as such you could gain more marks for your management of the problem than for pure factual knowledge. You are advised, therefore, to consider what you would **actually** do or wish to do in the given situation.

7 The available marks vary between one question and another; you are advised to work steadily through and not delay too long on any one question.

8 **Each page of the MEQ paper is marked independently. You should therefore answer each question specifically, even if this answer involves repetition of part of an earlier answer.**

9 As a rough guide, it is indicated when you have completed approximately one-third and two-thirds of each paper.

Harry Howes is a well known local character. His main claim to fame is that he has reared generations of champion racing pigeons. Harry is aged 50. He works as a furnace man in a local factory. He drinks heavily and admits to smoking 10 cigarettes a day. He has two daughters, one of whom is expecting her first baby. His wife is a timid woman whom you have seen frequently over the years with gynaecological and psychosomatic ailments. They appear happily married.

You rarely see Harry. The only note in your records is of a probable hiatus hernia, demonstrated on a barium meal three years ago. Harry comes to see you complaining of burning in his legs and feet for three months. His joints ache at the end of the day and at times he has been awakened by paraesthesiae in his hands and feet.

1 a) What are the three most likely diagnostic possibilities?

    b) What steps would you take at this consultation in order to clarify the diagnosis?

MEQ

Further elaboration of the history and physical examination do not reveal any more information. BP 155/90, urine — NAD. He is overweight and plethoric with a high colour.

2 a) What would you say to him?

   b) What further action would you take?

When you see him two weeks later the situation is unchanged, and your investigations have revealed no abnormality.

3   What would you do now?

MEQ

You treat him expectantly and follow him up. Several weeks later you notice definite signs of 'finger clubbing'.

4   Name the three most likely causes of clubbing in this patient.

YOU HAVE NOW COMPLETED APPROXIMATELY ONE-THIRD OF THE PAPER

Harry now complains of cough, breathlessness on exertion, and an ache in his left shoulder and upper chest. Examination reveals generalized expiratory rhonchi. He looks generally unwell.

5 a) What the three most likely causes of his chest condition?

   b) What further investigations are now indicated?

MEQ

Chest X-ray is reported as follows: 'There are signs of bronchopneumonic changes in the left upper lobe'. Sputum culture revealed *Haemophilus influenzae*, no malignant cells present. FBC normal, haemoglobin 16.1 g.

6 a) What is your assessment of the case now?

   b) What treatment, if any, would you prescribe and why?

He does not respond to your treatment, and he looks and feels worse. The cough is the most troublesome feature and he describes vertigo and faintness when he coughs. The chest signs are unchanged.

You decide to refer him urgently to a chest physician.

7   Write your referral letter below.

YOU HAVE NOW COMPLETED APPROXIMATELY TWO-THIRDS OF THE PAPER

MEQ

Harry is admitted to hospital for investigation. A few days later Mrs Howes and her two daughters come to see you in a very distressed and angry state. The specialist told them the previous night that he had cancer and there is not much that they can do for him.

8 a) How do you react to this situation?

   b) What would you say to the relatives?

Harry comes home to spend his last few weeks. He develops severe pain in his left hip due to bony metastases and he becomes increasingly short of breath.

9   a)   What further help can you offer?

    b)   What drugs would you prescribe for him and how would you advise administration?

MEQ

Harry dies 10 days later. Post-mortem shows a highly malignant carcinoma of the left upper lobe bronchus with secondaries in the mediastinal lymph nodes, the liver, the pancreas and the pericardium. The heart is enlarged with an area of old fibrosis in the left ventricle. The coronary arteries are arteriosclerotic.

10 What particular problems should you be prepared for with Mrs Howes during the next year and how might you forestall them?

THE ANSWERS TO MEQ TEST 1 APPEAR ON P 91

Gillian Frost is 12 years old. She is normally healthy and you have not seen her since the age of seven. Her father is a store manager and her mother works in an office. There are two younger brothers, aged eight and six years.

Her mother brings her to see you because one breast is larger than the other and feels a little tender. She has not yet started her periods.

1 a) What is the most likely cause of this problem?

    b) How would you explain the normal physical development of an adolescent girl to Gillian and her mother?

MEQ

Three years later Mrs Frost comes to see you. She is obviously in an anxious state and she tells you that she has just found out that Gillian has been missing from school frequently over the past few weeks.

2 a) What further questions would you ask Mrs Frost?

   b) What diagnostic term would you give to Gillian's behaviour?

   c) What other condition presents as absence from school and how does it differ from Gillian's problem?

62

Mrs Frost says that Gillian has been rebellious, sulky and moody at home. She stays out late at night and her parents disapprove of her friends. Previously she had done quite well at her school, the local comprehensive, but she now refuses to do any homework and has had bad reports.

3   How would you handle the situation?

YOU HAVE NOW COMPLETED APPROXIMATELY ONE-THIRD OF THE PAPER

MEQ

A few weeks later Gillian appears in the surgery by herself. She looks unwell and complains of a 'bad sore throat' for the past two days.

4 a) Give 3 likely and 2 possible causes for an acute sore throat in this age group.

Further elaboration of the history reveals no unusual features. On examination she has an acutely inflamed pharynx, tender, palpable cervical lymph nodes and a pyrexia of 100.4°F. Otherwise, there is nothing to find on examination.

   b) What investigations, if any, would you arrange? Give your reasons.

   c) Write out a prescription for Gillian. Justify each item.

She does not respond to your treatment and one week later you see her at home in bed. Her throat looks and feels worse, drinking is difficult and eating is impossible. She has widespread lymphadenopathy, a palpable liver and spleen and she is slightly jaundiced.

5   a) What is the most likely diagnosis now?

    b) How would you confirm this diagnosis?

    c) How would you manage the situation now?

MEQ

Gillian slowly recovers from her illness and goes back to school. Three months later you are just finishing a long evening surgery when the receptionist comes in to say that Mr and Mrs Frost are asking to see you straight away. Gillian is accompanying them.

6   How do you respond to this request? Explain your answer.

It transpires that her parents have learnt through a third party that Gillian's boyfriend has been referred to a VD clinic. In private, Gillian admits that she has been having intercourse with him but refuses absolutely to attend the clinic herself.

7   How would you manage this situation?

YOU HAVE NOW COMPLETED APPROXIMATELY TWO-THIRDS OF THE PAPER

All investigations are negative, with the exception of the pregnancy test which is positive. Gillian, now thoroughly chastened, comes back to see you with her mother one week later.

8   What areas would you want to explore in this consultation?

The family have already discussed the likelihood that Gillian was pregnant. It is now nearly eight weeks since her last menstrual period.
They request termination of the pregnancy.

9   a)   Under what circumstances is termination of pregnancy legal in the United Kingdom?

    b)   What action would you take?

MEQ

The pregnancy is terminated and post-operatively all goes well. Six weeks after the operation Gillian comes back to see you.

10 a) What is the purpose of a consultation at this stage.

b) How would you advise her?

THE ANSWERS TO MEQ TEST 2 APPEAR ON P 101

You have looked after Mrs Dawson during the antenatal period of her first pregnancy. She and her husband, who is a market gardener, live in a pleasant, privately owned house adjacent to their two acres of land. Both have been healthy and they are in their late twenties. There is no family history of note, apart from the maternal father who has 'always been chesty'. The pregnancy and birth were normal and Mrs Dawson takes a low-dose combined oral contraceptive. Jimmy has been attending children's clinic regularly. He is now four months old and bottle-fed. Mrs Dawson seeks your advice about the eczematous rash she has noted on Jimmy's face, antecubital fossa and popliteal areas.

1   a)   What is the most likely diagnosis?

    b)   What would you say to Mrs Dawson at this stage?

MEQ

You decide that he has atopic eczema.

2   a)   Write out a prescription for him. Justify each item.

    b)   How would you plan to manage this problem in the future?

The skin condition is well controlled by your management. Jimmy is now three years old and attends the local play group, which he enjoys. However, since starting he has suffered from constant coughs and colds.

One morning you are called to see him as an emergency. He has had a bad night with difficulty in breathing and a cough. He looks unwell and appears distressed, lying still and breathing rapidly. You can hear wheezing even before you place your stethoscope on his chest.

3   a)   What factors would you take into account in deciding whether or not to admit him to hospital?

    b)   If you decide to keep him at home what immediate treatment would you give him and why?

MEQ

Following this bout Jimmy becomes a frequent attender with recurrent coughs, colds and bouts of wheezing. Mrs Dawson states that he hardly eats anything, has difficulty in sleeping and is breathing badly. He is now four years old. She asks, 'Do you think perhaps he should have his tonsils out, doctor?'.

4   a)   How would you reply?

     b)   What further action would you take?

YOU HAVE NOW COMPLETED APPROXIMATELY ONE-THIRD OF THE PAPER

On further discussion it becomes apparent that there are problems with the marrriage. Mr Dawson has had more than one affair, the business is not doing well and they have financial problems.

5   What help can you offer to Mrs Dawson?

MEQ

The crisis resolves over the next few months and Jimmy starts school. His asthma is reasonably well controlled.
A year later Mrs Dawson comes to see you again. She complains of 'funny sensations like electric shocks' in her left arm, left leg and left side of her trunk for the past few days.

6 a) Suggest three possible causes for her symptoms?

   b) How would you seek to establish a diagnosis?

You do not find any objective abnormality and the neurologist to whom she is referred is unable to make a definite diagnosis. However, six months later she has an episode of retro-bulbar neuritis and hospital investigation suggests the likelihood of multiple sclerosis.
Mr and Mrs Dawson come to see you in surgery after her discharge from hospital. She has now fully recovered.

7   a)   How would you handle this consultation?

    b)   What areas would you want to cover in either this or subsequent consultations?

YOU HAVE NOW COMPLETED APPROXIMATELY TWO-THIRDS OF THE PAPER

MEQ

Jimmy's asthma has been quite well controlled for several years with intermittent oral bronchodilator therapy and antibiotics. However, he is now 10 years old and he finds it increasingly difficult to take part in games such as football because of shortness of breath. On two occasions he has required an injection to relieve an acute attack.

8 a) What general help and advice can you give to the family in respect of Jimmy's asthma?

   b) What specific prophylactic measures are available and how should they be administered?

Mr and Mrs Dawson come to see you together. Her last menstrual period had started seven weeks previously and she usually has a regular cycle. They have been using the sheath as a contraceptive method for several years but admit to occasional lapses. You are able to confirm at the time that Mrs Dawson is indeed seven weeks pregnant.

9   How would you advise them?

MEQ

Mrs Dawson keeps well during her pregnancy and is safely delivered of a full term, healthy baby girl. However, within three months of her delivery she has a serious relapse of her multiple sclerosis and develops specific weakness of her right arm and left leg, together with incontinence of urine. She becomes understandably depressed about her situation.

10   What can you do to help this patient and her family?

THE ANSWERS TO MEQ TEST 3 APPEAR ON P 108

Judith Blair is 19 years old. She has recently registered with you and lives with Sean Connery, aged 22 years, in a rented house. She is 26 weeks in her second pregnancy; her older child, Stephen, is nearly two. He was born before she met Sean.
She has been booked for delivery in the GP obstetric unit (24-hour stay). There is nothing significant in her previous medical history.
A home visit is requested because Judith suddenly developed a fever and started vomiting the previous evening.

1 a) What are the three most likely possible diagnoses?

   b) How would you differentiate between the various possibilities?

MEQ

You have good clinical reason to think that she has a urinary tract infection. Obstetric findings are all normal.

2   a)   Write a prescription for Judith. Justify each item.

      b)   What would be your further management of the situation?

The pregnancy continues satisfactorily until term and Judith is admitted in labour.
You are present at the delivery which is perfectly normal. Sean is not present. Unfortunately, however, the baby has an obvious meningomyelocoele.

3   a) How would you assess the degree of disability in the child?

    b) What would you say to the parents?

MEQ

You visit Judith in the maternity ward and find her weepy and depressed. Neither she nor Sean wish to have anything to do with the baby, John, who has been transferred to the neurosurgical unit 20 miles away for operation.

4 a) How would you handle this situation?

   b) What other professional workers would you expect to be involved? What would you expect them to do?

YOU HAVE NOW COMPLETED APPROXIMATELY ONE-THIRD OF THE PAPER

It is now ten weeks later. The baby, John, has undergone an operation to close the neural tube defect and hydrocephalus has not ensued. Two weeks ago he was transferred to the local paediatric unit. Judith has visited him twice in hospital and appears to accept him but Sean has refused to visit.
A case conference is arranged.

5 a) What is the purpose of this case conference?

   b) Who would you expect to be invited?

   c) If a decision is made that John should not return home, how could this be carried out and where might he go?

John eventually comes home at three months of age and appears to be doing well, although he has flaccid paralysis of the legs and is most unlikely ever to achieve continence. Judith brings him up to the surgery for a check-up and asks about immunisation. ·

6   How would you advise her?

At the same consultation, Judith tells you that she thinks she is pregnant again and admits that she has not been taking her contraceptive pills regularly. The pregnancy is subsequently confirmed.

A few weeks later, when John is almost six months old and Judith is about 14 weeks pregnant, she telephones you one evening in a panic and tells you that John was apparently well and taking his feeds normally when suddenly he stiffened, then 'shook all over' and 'his eyes rolled up in his head'.

7   a)   What is it about this call that makes you decide to visit right away?

   b)   What advice would you give her over the telephone?

YOU HAVE NOW COMPLETED APPROXIMATELY TWO-THIRDS OF THE PAPER

When you arrive a few minutes later he is sleepy but otherwise seems all right. Judith is alone in the house with him and Stephen aged two years.

8   a)   What further questions would you ask her?

     b)   What would you look for especially during your examination of John?

There is nothing significant in the history or on general examination. However, his pupils are well dilated and you are able to get a good view of his fundi which shows evidence of multiple small retinal haemorrhages.

9   a)   What is the significance of this finding?

b)   What would you say to Judith?

c)   What further action would you take?

MEQ

John is admitted to hospital for further care.

10   What are the common characteristics and circumstances of parents who harm their children?

THE ANSWERS TO MEQ TEST 4 APPEAR ON P 116

Answers

Harry Howes is a well known local character. His main claim to fame is that he has reared generations of champion racing pigeons.

Harry is aged 50. He works as a furnace man in a local factory. He drinks heavily and admits to smoking 10 cigarettes a day. He has two daughters, one of whom is expecting her first baby. His wife is a timid woman whom you have seen frequently over the years with gynaecological and psychosomatic ailments. They appear happily married.

You rarely see Harry. The only note in your records is of a probable hiatus hernia, demonstrated on a barium meal three years ago.

Harry comes to see you complaining of burning in his legs and feet for three months. His joints ache at the end of the day and at times he has been awakened by paraesthesiae in his hands and feet.

1 a) What are the three most likely diagnostic possibilities?

       Peripheral neuritis   — alcoholic
                            — diabetic
                            — associated with malignant disease
                            — industrial toxicity from factory   3%

       Other reasonable suggestions

  b) What steps would you take at this consultation in order to clarify the diagnosis?

       History   — alcohol intake, thirst, polyuria, weight, factory conditions (toxic substances), family history, systematic questions — cough, SOB, SOA, appetite, sleep, bowels, micturition, sex   3%

       Examination — full (may be deferred for a day or two if pressure of time)
                      — CVS, RS, AS, GUS
                      — special attention to CNS   { pain
                      — limbs — tone, power, reflexes, sensation { touch   3%
                                                   { temperature

       Investigation — urinalysis for sugar and albumen   2%

                                                  11% of total marks

MEQ

TP i) Marks would be awarded in relation to the relative likelihood of causes in general practice.
ii) Marks for brief, relevant history.
iii) Marks for precise, specific, relevant examination.
iv) Urinalysis is mandatory — likely to be marked highly.
v) Realities of general practice recognised.

Further elaboration of the history and physical examination do not reveal any more information. BP 155/90, urine — NAD.

He is overweight and plethoric with a high colour.

2   a) What would you say to him?

Explanation — impression of honesty
— plan of investigation   2%

Advice re. — alcohol intake
— weight control
— smoking   2%

Follow-up — see again, not more than 2 weeks   1%

b) What further action would you take?

Investigations — full blood count and film
— ESR
— random blood sugar
— serum gamma glutamyl transpeptidase
— liver function tests
— chest x-ray   3%

Contact factory doctor to exclude possibility of industrial toxicity   1%

9% of total marks

TP   i) No marks at this stage for SMA plus, SMA 12, serum B12 or folate levels.
      ii) Include investigations on this page even if noted in question 1.
          Remember each page of the examination MEQ is marked by different examiners.
          Therefore, comments such as 'see page 1' will *not* attract any marks.

When you see him 2 weeks later the situation is unchanged, and your investigations have revealed no abnormality.

3   What would you do now?

    1 Explanation — all tests normal
                    — often difficult problem to unravel   2%

    2 History   — recheck significant points
                    — explore sources of stress or anxiety   2%

    3 Examination — recheck peripheral nervous system   2%

    4 Advice   — wait and see
                    — offer possibility of referral
                    — continue encouragement to lose weight and reduce
                      alcohol intake   2%

8% of total marks

TP   The use of time as a diagnostic instrument in the absence of significant signs can be a
      reasonable option in general practice.

93

MEQ

You treat him expectantly and follow him up. Several weeks later you notice definite signs of 'finger clubbing'.

4   Name the three most likely causes of clubbing in this patient.

    1   Cirrhosis of the liver   1%

    2   Carcinoma of the bronchus   1%

    3   Extrinsic allergic alveolitis   1%

    4   Any other reasonable possibility

3% of total marks

TP   i) Keep an open mind!
          ii) Marks for purely factual knowledge are accorded low priority in MEQs.

Harry now complains of cough, breathlessness on exertion, and an ache in his left shoulder and upper chest. Examination reveals generalised expiratory rhonchi. He looks generally unwell.

5   a) What are the three most likely causes of his chest condition?

    1   Bronchitis   1%

    2   Extrinsic allergic alveolitis (bird fancier's lung)   1%

    3   Carcinoma of bronchus with secondary infection   1%

    4   Any other reasonable suggestion (as an alternative)

b) What further investigations are now indicated?

    1   Repeat chest x-ray — PA and left lateral views   2%

    2   Peak-flow or vitallograph   1%

    3   Sputum examination for — culture
                               — eosinophils
                               — cytology   1%

    4   Repeat full blood count   1%

                                            8% of total marks

TP   Remember the pigeons!

Chest x-ray is reported as follows: 'There are signs of bronchopneumonic changes in the left upper lobe'. Sputum culture revealed *Haemophilus influenzae*, no malignant cells present. FBC normal, haemoglobin 16.1 g.

6   a)   What is your assessment of the case now?

    1   Chest infection which requires treatment   1%

    2   Chest infection does *not* explain clubbing   2%

    3   Negative sputum cytology does *not* exclude malignancy   2%

    4   Carcinoma of bronchus must be excluded   2%

                                            95

MEQ

b) What treatment, if any, would you prescribe and why?

1 Broad spectum antibiotic — to eradicate pathogens

    either   ampicillin 250 to 500 mg qds
    or   amoxycillin 250 mg tds
    or   co-trimoxazole 2 tabs bd
    or   oxytetracycline 250 to 500 mg qds

    may be guided by sputum report but often unreliable

    other reasons — cost, bioavailability, side-effects, etc.   3%

2 Antispasmodic — to relieve bronchospasm

    either β-sympathomimetic drug orally or by
             inhalation, e.g. salbutamol, orciprenaline
    or   theophylline orally
    or   acceptable alternative

    other reasons — cost, bioavailability, side-effects, etc.   1%

3 Mild analgesic — to relieve pain
                  — avoid aspirin (hiatus hernia)   1%

                          12% of total marks

TP   i) Write down positive and negative points.
       ii) Note dosage and route of administration where applicable.

He does not respond to your treatment, and looks and feels worse. The cough is the most troublesome feature and he describes vertigo and faintness when he coughs. The chest signs are unchanged.
    You decide to refer him urgently to a chest physician.

96

7   Write your referral letter below.

General information	— urgency of appointment — date of birth — home circumstances — occupation — hobbies (pigeon-fancier)	2%
Past medical history	— smoking habits — drinking habits — hiatus hernia	2%
Events leading to referral	— description of condition — GP's findings — results of investigations — GP's opinion	2%
Management	— drug treatment — information given to patient — information given to wife	2%
Request to consultant	— arrange further investigations — advise on treatment — offer to assist and continue — care as required	2%

10% of total marks

TP   Few referral letters contain all the information which may be useful to the consultant.

Harry is admitted to hospital for investigation. A few days later Mrs Howes and her two daughters come to see you in a very distressed and angry state. The specialist told them the previous night that he had cancer and there is not much that they can do for him.

8 a) How do you react to this situation?

Avoid confrontation	1%
Allow ventilation of feelings	1%
Express sympathy and concern	1%
Seek more information and confirmation of diagnosis	1%
Later: Check completeness of medical record	1%
Discuss case with Defence Union if anxious	1%

b) What would you say to the relatives?

Explanation of — diagnosis	1%
— prognosis	1%
— therapy available	1%
— care available from primary health care team and other services	1%
Exploration of — feelings of anger, grief, anxiety, distress	2%

12% of total marks

TP Try to think yourself into the situation and analyse how you would react. Write down how you would behave as well as what you would say and do.

Harry comes home to spend his last few weeks. He develops severe pain in his left hip due to bony metastases and he becomes increasingly short of breath.

98

9   a)   What further help can you offer?

Review contribution of primary health care team	1%
Review home conditions and ability of wife to cope	1%
Consider admission to hospice or hospital	1%
Consider palliative radiotherapy	1%
Consider oxygen therapy	1%
Provide support and counselling	1%
Continue regular visiting	1%

b)   What drugs would you prescribe for him and how would you advise administration?

1   Give drugs to anticipate pain   1%

2   Use a hierarchy of agents and dosage   1%

3   Moderate analgesics — in correct dosage
    — oral, e.g. dihydrocodeine, phenazoline, dextromoramide   1%

4   Strong analgesics — in correct dosage
    — oral, e.g. 'Brompton Cocktail'
        or   mist. diamorph., cocaine + chlorpromazine BNF
        or   mist. morph. + phenothiazine   2%

    — parenteral, e.g. diamorph. + phenothiazine
                or   Cyclimorph   1%

    — suppository, e.g. Palflum
                or   Proladone   1%

5   Management of constipation
        e.g. fluids, bran, Dorbanex, etc.   1%

15% of total marks

TP   i) Try to provide a broad range of alternative strategies.
      ii) Pay attention to detail.

Harry dies 10 days later. Post-mortem shows a highly malignant carcinoma of the left upper lobe bronchus with secondaries in the mediastinal lymph nodes, the liver, the pancreas and the pericardium. The heart is enlarged with an area of old fibrosis in the left ventricle. The coronary arteries are arteriosclerotic.

10 What particular problems should you be prepared for with Mrs Howes during the next year and how might you forestall them?

1   Increased risk of physical and mental illness including suicide   2%

2   Stages of bereavement — shock, numbness, inability to accept
                     — anger, blame — herself
                                     — family
                                     — GP
                                     — others
                     — realisation and hopelessness
                     — gradual acceptance and recovery
                     — outline of usual time-scale   4%

3   Unlikely possibility of litigation or complaint   1%

4   See regularly   — support, counselling, ventilation of feelings
                       — stress inevitability of death
                       — stress irrelevance of early diagnosis in carcinoma of lung
                       — stress her great value to husband, praise her efforts,
                          encourage outside activities when appropriate   4%

5   Use contacts with other family members to provide indirect support   1%

12% of total marks

TP   Think around the situation as it might occur in your practice and write down how you would actually handle it.

Answers

Gillian Frost is 12 years old. She is normally healthy and you have not seen her since the age of 7. Her father is a store manager and her mother works in an office. There are two younger brothers, aged 8 and 6 years.

Her mother brings her to see you because one breast is larger than the other and feels a little tender. She has not yet started her periods.

1 a) What is the most likely cause of this problem?

      Pubertal mastitis   1%

   b) How would you explain the normal physical development of an adolescent girl to Gillian and her mother?

      1 Hormones in the body are starting to change her from a girl into a woman 1%
      2 Breast development is usually the first sign of puberty.   1%
      3 Breast development is often unequal at first.   1%
      4 Breast tenderness is common and not serious:
         It will settle in time.   1%
      5 Pubic and axillary hair will appear later.   1%
      6 Periods start on average about two years after the first
         signs of breast development.   1%
      7 It takes several years to complete the whole process and periods
         may be heavy and irregular at first.   1%

                                         8% of total marks

TP   Remember to present information clearly and in a logical sequence.

Three years later Mrs Frost comes to see you. She is obviously in an anxious state and she tells you that she has just found out that Gillian has been missing from school frequently over the past few weeks.

MEQ

2 a) What further questions would you ask Mrs Frost?

     1 How did she find out about it?   1%

     2 How does Gillian relate to the family and friends?   1%

     3 How has Gillian been behaving in general recently   1%
        ?sleep ?appetite ?mood swings ?enuresis   1%

     4 Any major life-events in family, e.g. death, illness,
        marital discord?   1%

     5 What was Gillian's school record previously?   1%

     6 What does Mrs Frost think is the cause of Gillian's
        behaviour?   1%

  b) What diagnostic term would you give to Gillian's behaviour?

     Truancy   1%

  c) What other condition presents as absence from school and how does it differ from Gillian's problem?

     School phobia — due to separation anxiety
                — complex overdependent mother/child relationship
                — occurs equally in both sexes
                — affects younger children, often 9 to 12 years
                — requires skilled help (GP ± psychiatric services)
                   to restart school attendance and deal with family
                   problems   4%

     Truancy   — usually teenagers
                — often socially determined, peer-group behaviour
                — often indicator of other associated problems,
                   e.g. educational, emotional
                — responsibility of Education Welfare Service   4%

16% of total marks

TP   Large question. Should be a TEQ!

Mrs Frost says that Gillian has been rebellious, sulky and moody at home. She stays out late at night and her parents disapprove of her friends. Previously she had done quite well at her school, the local comprehensive, but she now refuses to do any homework and has had bad reports.

3   How would you handle the situation?

    1   Listen sympathetically.   1%

    2   Offer help and support.   1%

    3   Advise re nature of condition.   1%

    4   Identify problem areas.   1%

    5   Advise parents to contact Headmaster.   1%

    6   Offer to see Gillian if she wants to see you,
but stress that you are not able to do anything
directly unless she is prepared to see you.   2%

    7% of total marks

TP   Think around the problem. Include ethical dilemmas where appropriate.

A few weeks later Gillian appears in the surgery by herself. She looks unwell and complains of a 'bad sore throat' for the past two days.

4   a)   Give three likely and two possible causes for an acute sore throat in this age group.

    1   a)   Viral pharyngitis   1%

        b)   Streptococcal pharyngitis   1%

        c)   Glandular fever   1%

    2   a)   Blood dyscrasia, e.g. leukaemia with secondary infection   1%

        b)   Gonococcal pharyngitis   1%

  or c)   Any other reasonable suggestion (as an alternative).

Further elaboration of the history reveals no unusual features. On examination she has an acutely inflamed pharynx, tender, palpable cervical lymph nodes and a pyrexia of 100.4°F. Otherwise there is nothing to find on examination.

    b)   What investigations, if any, would you arrange? Give your reasons.

        NIL — no clinical evidence of any serious condition
            — saving of resources
            — no harm done by expectant policy   2%

103

MEQ

    c) Write out a prescription for Gillian. Justify each item.

        1 Soluble aspirin or paracetamol
               2 tabs qds. ac: — for pain and pyrexia
                                — best used as a gargle   1%

        2 Penicillin V 250 mg qds orally — cheap
           for at least 5 days   — effective against streps
           (Phenethicillin acceptable as alternative)   2%

                                      10% of total marks

TP   i) Investigation not usual at this stage in UK.
        ii) Aspirin or paracetamol may well be advised rather than prescribed.
      iii) Ampicillin or Amoxil *not* acceptable due to risk of florid rash in glandular fever.
      iv) Other antibiotics *not* acceptable on grounds of cost, efficacy, etc.

She does not respond to your treatment and one week later you see her at home in bed. Her throat looks and feels worse, drinking is difficult and eating is impossible. She has widespread lymphadenopathy, a palpable liver and spleen and she is slightly jaundiced.

5   a) What is the most likely diagnosis now?

          Glandular fever   1%

    b) How would you confirm this diagnosis?

        1 Throat swab — to exclude pathogenic bacteria   1%

        2 Full blood count — for atypical monocytes and relative
           lymphocytosis   1%

        3 Paul Bunnell or Monospot test — should be positive at this
           stage if due to Epstein—Barr virus glandular fever   1%

        4 SMA 12 to assess liver function   1%

    c) How would you manage the situation now?

        1 Explain diagnosis and management to family   1%

        2 Stress good prognosis, no specific treatment   1%

        3 Advise rest, stronger analgesics if required, adequate
           fluid intake   1%

    4 Hospitalization not indicated; offer domiciliary
      consultation if doctor or parents anxious   1%
    5 Follow up carefully (self or practice nurse)   1%
    6 Advise parents to contact you if anxious.   1%

                                     11% of total marks

TP   Include reasons for investigations ordered.

Gillian slowly recovers from her illness and goes back to school. Three months later you are just finishing a long evening surgery when the receptionist comes in to say that Mr and Mrs Frost are asking to see you straight away. Gillian is accompanying them.

6   How do you respond to this request? Explain your answer.

      1 Probably suppressed irritation   1%
      2 See them at end of surgery — family and background known   2%
                                 — likely to be some type of psychosocial
                                    crisis — both parents!   2%
                                      — unlikely that another doctor, e.g.
                                      partner or relief service doctor,
                                      could handle situation as well   2%

                                        7% of total marks

TP   Honesty is the best policy!

It transpires that her parents have learnt through a third party that Gillian's boyfriend has been referred to a VD clinic. In private, Gillian admits that she has been having intercourse with him but refuses absolutely to attend the clinic herself.

7   How would you manage this situation?

      1 Offer non-judgemental sympathy and support   1%
      2 Try to contact VD clinic for details of boyfriend's condition   1%
      3 Explain risks of VD   1%

                                          105

Then, either at the time or within the next day or two:

4   Try again to persuade her to attend the clinic if indicated.
    If unsuccessful....   1%
5   Take a gynaecological history — including other sexual contacts   1%
6   General examination   1%
7   Gynaecological exam — send charcoal swabs in transport medium
                         — from cervix, urethra, rectum and pharynx
                         — HVS for culture
                         — cervical smear for cytology
                         — blood for serology
                         — pregnancy test   3%
8   Treat appropriately — with advice from specialist if required   1%
9   Arrange follow-up and contraceptive advice   1%

                                                            11% of total marks

TP   i) Again, try and think yourself into the situation.
    ii) Include physical, psychological and social factors.

All investigations are negative, with the exception of the pregnancy test which is positive. Gillian, now thoroughly chastened, comes back to see you with her mother one week later.

8   What areas would you want to explore in this consultation?

        1 Attitudes to pregnancy   — Gillian
                                      — boyfriend
                                      — mother and family   2%
        2 Attitudes to termination — emotional
                                      — religious
                                      — legal   2%
        3 Attitudes to adoption   2%
        4 Present relationship with boyfriend   2%
        5 Future expectations — marriage
                               — school
                               — career   2%

                                                            10% of total marks

TP You are asked what areas you would want to explore, *not* how would you manage this situation in terms of action. Read the question!

The family have already discussed the likelihood that Gillian was pregnant. It is now nearly eight weeks since her last menstrual period.
They request termination of the pregnancy.

9 a) Under what circumstances is termination of pregnancy legal in the United Kingdom?

The continuance of pregnancy would involve:

1 Risk to the life of the pregnant woman greater than if the pregnancy were terminated.   2%

2 Risk of injury to the physical or mental health of the pregnant woman greater than if the pregnancy were terminated   2%

3 Risk of injury to the physical or mental health of the existing children of the family of the pregnant woman greater than if the pregnancy were terminated.   2%

4 There is substantial risk that if the child were born it would suffer from such physical or mental abnormalities as to be severely handicapped.   2%

b) What action would you take?

Either — referral to gynaecologist.
or   — referral to BPAS or similar.
or   — referral to another colleague for opinion.   2%

10% of total marks

TP i) See Green Form
    ii) In (b) a blank refusal is not acceptable even if the doctor has strong religious convictions. The patient must be offered the opportunity to consult another practitioner, either a GP, or specialist.

The pregnancy is terminated and post-operatively all goes well. Six weeks after the operation Gillian comes back to see you.

10 a) What is the purpose of a consultation at this stage?

       1 Assess − physical state
                − psychological state
                − social state   2%

       2 Consider contraception   2%

       3 Allow time for discussion on any topic Gillian may want to raise   2%

  b) How would you advise her?

       1 Risks associated with repeated termination   1%

       2 Need for contraception − in most cases even if 'not required' at present   1%

       3 Discuss alternative methods   1%

       4 Stress availability in case of future crisis   1%

10% of total marks

TP   Remember to mention leaving space for patient's problems and offer availability.

MEQ
TEST 3

Answers

You have looked after Mrs Dawson during the antenatal period of her first pregnancy. She and her husband, who is a market gardener, live in a pleasant, privately owned house adjacent to their two acres of land. Both have been healthy and they are in their late twenties. There is no family history of note, apart from the maternal father who has 'always been chesty'. The pregnancy and birth were normal and Mrs Dawson takes a low-dose combined oral contraceptive. Jimmy has been attending children's clinic regularly. He is now four months old and bottle-fed. Mrs Dawson seeks your advice about the eczematous rash she has noted on Jimmy's face, antecubital fossa and popliteal areas.

1 a) What is the most likely diagnosis?

       Infantile eczema − probably atopic   1%

b) What would you say to Mrs Dawson at this stage?

Explanation	– common problem, can be relieved but not cured, usually resolves spontaneously	2%
Advice	– use bath oil, aqueous cream or other soap substitute	
	– apply cream (½ per cent hydrocortisone) thinly on affected areas twice a day	
	– keep mittens on hands	3%
Follow-up	– see 1 to 2 weeks	1%

7% of total marks

TP   Follow logical order – explanation, advice, arrangements for follow-up.

You decide that he has atopic eczema.

2 a) Write out a prescription for him. Justify each item.

1	Hydrocortisone cream ½ per cent 30 g	– anti-inflammatory	
	Sig . . apply bd.	– anti-pruritic	
		– safe	
		– cheap	2%
2	Aqueous cream BP 200 g	– soothing	
	Sig . . use as soap substitute	– emollient	
		– safe	
		– cheap	2%

b) How would you plan to manage this problem in the future?

1	Support and advise parents	1%
2	Monitor progress of eczema at regular intervals	1%
3	Use soap substitute for prolonged period	1%
4	Use steroid cream intermittently if possible	1%
5	Consider referral if deterioration of condition	1%

9% of total marks

TP   Emphasise effective, proven, safe, cheap drugs from BNF if possible.

MEQ

The skin condition is well controlled by your management. Jimmy is now three years old and attends the local play group, which he enjoys. However, since starting he has suffered from constant coughs and colds.

One morning you are called to see him as an emergency. He has had a bad night with difficulty in breathing and a cough. He looks unwell and appears distressed, lying still and breathing rapidly. You can hear wheezing even before you place your stethoscope on his chest.

3 a) What factors would you take into account in deciding whether or not to admit him to hospital?

    1   Degree of distress — child and parents   1%

    2   Cyanosis   1%

    3   Tachycardia 120/min or more   1%

    4   Intercostal recession and the use of auxiliary respiratory muscles   1%

    5   Response to presence and initial treatment   1%

    6   Home and transport facilities   1%

    b) If you decide to keep him at home what immediate treatment would you give him and why?

    Adrenaline 1 in 1000 solution (or alternative sympathomimetic)   1%
        — up to 0.5 ml slowly subcutaneously whilst
           monitoring pulse rate   1%
        — easy to administer, safe if careful, often
           effective   1%
    and/or Aminophylline 50 to 100 mg intravenously slowly   1%
        — effective, may be difficult to administer   1%

11% of total marks

TP   i) Three-year-old unlikely to use inhaler properly — although salbutamol could be tried.
    ii) Steroids unlikely to be necessary at this stage and do not have immediate action even if administered intravenously.

Following this bout Jimmy becomes a frequent attender with recurrent coughs, colds and bouts of wheezing. Mrs Dawson states that he hardly eats anything, has difficulty in sleeping and is breathing badly. He is now four years old. She asks, 'Do you think perhaps he should have his tonsils out, Doctor?''.

4   a)   How would you reply?

Open-ended questions	– how do you think it would help?	1%
	– are you finding it difficult to cope? Any other problems?	1%
Specific answers	– no evidence of recurrent tonsillitis	1%
	– no evidence that removing tonsils reduces rate of URTI or wheezy attacks	1%
	– explain risks of operation	1%
	– advise on good prognosis of 'catarrhal children'	1%
	– advise against operation	1%

b)   What further action would you take?

1   If advice accepted overtly and confirmed by demeanour
     – no further action   2%

2   If advice rejected verbally or if patient obviously unhappy
     – referral for second opinion   1%
     – paediatrician rather than surgeon   1%
     – preferably specialist whose views are known to you   1%

12% of total marks

TP   i)   Why did mother raise this question at this moment? Be aware of the covert content of the consultation.
      ii)   Note emphasis in (b) on non-verbal communication.

On further discussion it becomes apparent that there are problems with the marriage. Mr Dawson has had more than one affair, the business is not doing well and they have financial problems.

MEQ

5   What help can you offer to Mrs Dawson?

                Sympathy and support.   2%
                Availability.   2%
                Opportunity to talk.   2%
                Advice and help via   — health visitor.
                                       — social worker.
                                       — marriage guidance.
                                       — solicitor.   2%

                                                                    8% of total marks

TP   Help consists of what you can offer yourself and what other resources you may
        mobilise.

The crisis resolves over the next few months and Jimmy starts school. His asthma is reasonably well controlled.
A year later Mrs Dawson comes to see you again. She complains of 'funny sensations, like
electric shocks' in her left arm, left leg and left side of her trunk, for the past few days.

6   a) Suggest three possible causes for her symptoms

        1   Anxiety state   1%
        2   Migraine   1%
        3   Neurological disorder, e.g. multiple sclerosis   1%

     b) How would you seek to establish a diagnosis?

            History   — past episodes, any familial background
                       — present ?associated symptoms
                         present ?stress — physical or psychological
                       — general systematic questioning   3%
            Examination — general
                         — CNS — fundi
                                — limb tone, power and weakness
                                — sensation to touch, pinprick, temperature
                                  ? any difference between R and L sides
                                — test urine for sugar, protein   3%

Referral — if no positive evidence of migraine or anxiety or if
abnormal findings on examination   2%

11% of total marks

TP Marks for specific points of history and relevant examination.

You do not find any objective abnormality and the neurologist to whom she is referred is unable to make a definite diagnosis. However, six months later she has an episode of retro-bulbar neuritis and hospital investigation suggests the likelihood of multiple sclerosis.
Mr and Mrs Dawson come to see you in surgery after her discharge from hospital. She has now fully recovered.

7 a) How would you handle this consultation?

1 Find out what they know already about the diagnosis and prognosis   1%

2 Explain and clarify the present position   1%

3 Be guarded about prognosis   1%

4 Assure continuing help, support and provision of treatment if required 1%

b) What areas would you want to cover in either this or subsequent consultations?

1 Knowledge of disease and prognosis   1%

2 Marriage   1%

3 Difficulties with housework or employment outside of home   1%

4 Effects on child   1%

5 Any other areas of concern   1%

9% of total marks

TP Question 7a asks for details of how you would handle the process of this first consultation, whilst 7b asks about the content of this and subsequent consultations.

113

MEQ

Jimmy's asthma has been quite well controlled for several years with intermittent oral bronchodilator therapy and antibiotics. However, he is now 10 years old and he finds it increasingly difficult to take part in games such as football because of shortness of breath. On two occasions he has required an injection to relieve an acute attack.

8 a) What general help and advice can you give to the family in respect of Jimmy's asthma?

Reconsideration of possible trigger factors in addition to exercise	
– housedust, food, emotional stress, pets, etc.	1%
– removal of triggers if possible	1%
– consideration of desensitization (rarely effective)	1%
Encouragement to lead a normal life as far as possible	1%
Advice re. specific prophylactic measures	1%
Monitoring of severity by serial peak-flow readings	1%

b) What specific prophylactic measures are available and how should they be administered?

1 Disodium cromoglycate (Intal) by inhalation (spinhaler) qds is highly effective   1%

2 Salbutamol (Ventolin) by inhalation immediately before exercise   1%

3 Steroids aerosols by inhalation are effective and much safer than oral steroids   1%

4 Oral steroids are effective but not safe for prolonged use in children due to side-effects, especially stunting of growth. Severe cases may require this treatment but specialist guidance is advisable   1%

10% of total marks

TP   Range widely in questions of this type.

Mr and Mrs Dawson come to see you together. Her last menstrual period had started seven weeks previously and she usually has a regular cycle. They have been using the sheath as a contraceptive method for several years but admit to occasional lapses. You are able to confirm at the time that Mrs Dawson is indeed seven weeks pregnant.

9   How would you advise them?

    1   Pregnancy is confirmed, EDD   1%

    2   No increased risk to baby because of mother's condition   1%

    3   Increased risk of exacerbation of multiple sclerosis occurring either during pregnancy or in puerperium   2%

    4   Termination of the pregnancy would be legal under the Abortion Act and probably available under the NHS   1%

    5   The decision must be for the couple to take together   1%

    6   Preferably go away and think about it before coming to a decision   1%

    7   Come back next week – stress importance of not leaving a decision too late if they decide on termination   1%

    8   Offer continuing advice and support whatever decision they come to   1%

9% of total marks

TP   Be logical and concise and remember to think in physical, psychological and social terms.

Mrs Dawson keeps well during her pregnancy and is safely delivered of a full term, healthy baby girl. However, within three months of the delivery she has a serious relapse of her multiple sclerosis and develops specific weakness of her right arm and left leg, together with incontinence of urine. She becomes understandably depressed about her situation.

10   What can you do to help this patient and her family?

    1   Continuing sympathy and support, availability, allow time and opportunity for problems to be raised, anxieties aired and grief expressed   2%

    2   Liaise with health visitor re care of baby, provision of aid and local support, baby-minding, later playgroup facilities   2%

    3   Liaise with district nurse re nursing care, coping with incontinence   2%

    4   Liaise with social services re home help, casework, financial or employment problems, housing problems including modification or transfer   2%

5   Consider prescribing tricyclic antidepressant for (1) depression and
    (2) may help incontinence due to parasympatheticolytic action   2%

6   Consider prescribing ACTH injections or other drugs on specialist
    advice   2%

7   Monitor situation at frequent intervals.   2%

14% of total marks

TP   This type of question tests your ability to make plans and foresee problems.

MEQ
TEST 4

Answers

Judith Blair is 19 years old. She has recently registered with you and lives with Sean Connery, aged 22 years, in a rented house. She is 26 weeks in her second pregnancy; her older child, Stephen, is nearly two. He was born before she met Sean.
She has been booked for delivery in the GP obstetric unit (24 hour stay). There is nothing significant in her previous medical history.
A home visit is requested because Judith suddenly developed a fever and started vomiting the previous evening.

1   a)   What are the three most likely possible diagnoses?

     1   Urinary tract infection   1%

     2   'Gastric flu', 'virus gastritis', 'food poisoning'   1%

     3   Complication of pregnancy, e.g. hyperemesis   1%

    b)   How would you differentiate between the various possibilities?

     1   History   — past — any similar episodes, any serious illnesses,
                                  any allergies

         — present — food, drink, travel
                — associated symptoms, e.g. urinary, diarrhoea, headache
                — any vaginal bleeding   3%

2 Examination — general (T,P,R, jaundice, anaemia, glands)
                     — upper respiratory tract
                     — CNS (especially neck stiffness)
                     — CVS (especially BP)
                     — GUS (tenderness — loin or suprapubic, uterus — size, tenderness)
                     — AS (tenderness, guarding, rigidity)   3%

3 Investigation — MSU   1%

                                           10% of total marks

TP   Consider frequency of conditions presenting in general practice, not in hospital practice.

You have good clinical reason to think that she has a urinary tract infection. Obstetric findings are all normal.

2 a) Write a prescription for Judith. Justify each item.

       1   Caps amoxycillin 250 mg tds for one week
       or caps ampicillin 250 to 500 mg qds for one week
       or tabs Septrin 2 bd for one week   2%

       2   Antibiotic spectrum — likely pathogens
           Lack of teratogenicity or other side-effects
           Bio-availability
           Cost   2%

       3   Paracetamol 2 tabs prn   1%

  b) What would be your further management of the situation?

        Immediate   — rest, fluids, explanation of illness
                       — ?working, ?NHS cert.
                       — ?care of child — husband, other   2%

Later — follow-up, clinical and repeat MSU
— change antibiotics if indicated
— ?hospital admission if no improvement
— consider IVP in puerperium   3%

10% of total marks

TP   Try to put yourself in the situation and think about all the points you would consider.

The pregnancy continues satisfactorily until term and Judith is admitted in labour.
You are present at the delivery which is perfectly normal. Sean is not present. Unfortunately, however, the baby has an obvious meningomyelocoele.

3   a)   How would you assess the degree of disability in the child?

1	General appearance and condition	1%
2	Head shape and circumference	1%
3	Size and position of neural tube defect	1%
4	?Spontaneous movement of lower limbs	1%
5	?Reflex movement of lower limbs	1%
6	?Fixed deformity of lower limbs, e.g. talipes	1%

b)   What would you say to the parents?

Immediately — tell Judith the baby has a problem which will need
                       further investigation and treatment   2%
Soon   — try to see parents together   1%
               — explain nature of disability and future plans   1%
               — allow ventilation of — grief
                                                — anger
                                                — anxiety
                                                — guilt   1%
               — demonstrate sympathy and assure long-term help
                 and support   1%

12% of total marks

TP   In (b) think in terms of immediate and later management.

You visit Judith in the maternity ward and find her weepy and depressed. Neither she nor Sean wish to have anything to do with the baby, John, who has been transferred to the Neurosurgical unit 20 miles away for operation.

4   a) How would you handle this situation?

Immediate acceptance of feelings — stress not uncommon, may feel differently later on	2%
Liaise with district midwife, health visitor and social worker	1%
Arrange return home as soon as convenient	1%

    b) What other professional workers would you expect to be involved? What would you expect them to do?

District midwife	— routine postnatal care	
	— support and listening	1%
Health visitor	— support and counselling	
and/or	— advising re facilities for handicap, help available	
social worker	— work towards reconciling parents to accept and care for child	2%

7% of total marks

TP   Consider patient's reaction and skills of other workers.

It is now ten weeks later. The baby, John, has undergone an operation to close the neural tube defect and hydrocephalus has not ensued. Two weeks ago he was transferred to the local paediatric unit. Judith has visited him twice in hospital and appears to accept him but Sean has refused to visit.
A case conference is arranged.

MEQ

5 a) What is the purpose of this case conference?

      1 Alert relevant people, share knowledge and establish facts   1%

      2 Make a diagnosis in physical, psychological and social terms   1%

      3 Decide on care of John. ?care proceedings or place of safety order   1%

      4 Decide on plan for rest of family   1%

      5 Decide roles and responsibilities of the extended team   1%

b) Who would you expect to be invited?

      GP, health visitor, senior nursing officer, hospital social worker, community social worker, senior social worker, paediatrician, ward sister, paediatric SHO or HP, community physician, educational psychologist, parents   2%

c) If a decision is made that John should not return home, how could this be carried out and where might he go?

      1 Voluntarily   1%

      2 Place of Safety Order — if urgent
         Application by S/W signed by magistrate/sheriff, valid 28 days   1%

      3 Care Order — if not urgent
         Application by S/W to magistrates court, valid indefinitely   1%

      4 Stay in hospital   at discretion of   1%
         Go to foster-home   social services   1%
         Go to residential childrens home   1%

13% of total marks

TP   Some knowledge of the working of Social Services departments, and the legal framework within which they operate, is essential.

John eventually comes home at three months of age and appears to be doing well, although he has flaccid paralysis of the legs and is most unlikely ever to achieve continence. Judith brings him up to the surgery for a check-up and asks about immunisation.

6   How would you advise her?

General   — requires prophylactic immunisation even more than
            a normal child because more likely to develop compli-
            cations. However, some vaccines are contraindicated.   2%
Specific   — diptheria and tetanus — at normal intervals   1%
            — pertussis — contraindicated   1%
            — measles — at usual time   1%
            — small pox — contraindicated for all children now   1%
            — tuberculosis — later if required   1%

7% of total marks

TP   Straightforward question.

At the same consultation Judith tells you that she thinks she is pregnant again and admits that she has not been taking her contraceptive pill regularly. The pregnancy is subsequently confirmed.
A few weeks later, when John is almost six months old and Judith is about 14 weeks pregnant, she telephones you one evening in a panic and tells you that John was apparently well and taking his feeds normally when suddenly he stiffened, then 'shook all over' and 'his eyes rolled up in his head'.

7   a)   What is it about this call that makes you decide to visit right away?

1 Knowledge of previous history   1%
2 Sounds like possible convulsion or other serious condition   1%
3 Judith is frightened and in a panic   1%

b)   What advice would you give her over the telephone?

1 Not to panic — looks alarming but will soon stop   1%
2 Will come immediately   1%
3 Do not attempt to impede baby's movements
4 Do not interfere with mouth or clothes   1%

121

MEQ

5 Do not attempt to feed

6 Leave him on his side or on front on her knee or in cot,
not on his back   1%

7% of total marks

TP   Telephone medicine is an important facet of general practice.

When you arrive a few minutes later he is sleepy but otherwise seems alright. Judith is alone in the house with him and Stephen aged 2 years.

8   a)   What further questions would you ask her?

1   Ever had a similar episode?   1%

2   Any previous symptoms that day?   1%

3   Repeat detailed description of attack — before, during after   1%

4   Any family history of convulsions?   1%

b)   What would you look for especially during your examination of John?

1 Temperature   1%

2 General condition — colour, breathing, dehydration   1%

3 Common causes of febrile convulsion — otitis media,
pharyngitis, chest infection   1%

4 Evidence of meningitis — neck stiffness, tense fontanelle   1%

5 Evidence of trauma — bruises, bites, scalds, burns, fractures,
retinal haemorrhages   1%

9% of total marks

TP   Think of the likely conditions and how you would try to exclude them.

There is nothing significant in the history or on general examination. However, his pupils are well dilated and you are able to get a good view of his fundi which show evidence of multiple small retinal haemorrhages.

9 a) What is the significance of this finding?

        Evidence of injury caused by violent shaking of child   2%

    b) What would you say to Judith?

Explanation	– probably a fit, quite common	1%
Reassurance	– not usually of serious significance	1%
Reassess history	– gently inquire re circumstances again	1%
Advice	– best to admit to hospital	1%
	– requires observation	
	nursing care	
	further investigation	1%

    c) What further action would you take?

Contact paediatrician	1%
Arrange hospital admission	1%
Inform – partners, health visitor, social services	1%
Record detailed notes – may be required at case	
conference or legal proceedings	1%
Maintain close contact with family	1%

                                          12% of total marks

TP   Try to demonstrate tactful handling of a difficult situation.

John is admitted to hospital for further care.

10   What are the common characteristics and circumstances of parents who harm their children?

Personality/psychiatric features	— immaturity	
	— low tolerance of stress	
	— high usage of alcohol/drugs	
	— poor relationships with other adults	
	— anxiety/depression common	
	— psychopathy or psychosis more common than in general population	4%
Social features	— early marriage, pregnant before marriage, unplanned pregnancy, unwanted child	
	— poor bonding (prematurity, handicap, separation at birth)	
	— subjected to violence themselves as children	
	— own parents alcoholic	
	— social deprivation — poor housing, financial problems, overcrowding, more often in low social class	
	— lack of extended family support, rootless	
	— behaviour of child, e.g. miserable, crying	
	— marital problems	6%
Behaviour	— slow to report to medical services	
	— unconvincing explanation re injuries	
	— under stress	3%

13% of total marks

TP   Long question — should be a TEQ!

Traditional Essay Question or TEQ

There is a tendency to spend a great deal of time and effort on preparation for the multiple choice and modified essay sections of this examination at the expense of the traditional essay questions. The TEQ carries marks equal to those awarded for the other two sections and for this reason, if for no other, an equal amount of thought and energy should be devoted to it. Although it now receives less emphasis at all stages of the medical school curriculum, and the contemporary candidate is therefore perhaps less practised in its presentation than were his predecessors, it remains one of the best methods of assessing the doctor's ability to think logically, show his knowledge in its best possible light and present it clearly and succinctly.

The areas of general practice which the examination may cover include clinical, psychosocial and therapeutic aspects of disease as well as organisational matters and topics of current interest or controversy. While by no means invariable, it is often true that each of the three questions in one examination will be drawn from a different one of the groups. Thus the first question might be concerned with a clinical topic (hypertension, diabetes), while the second might deal with practice organisation (screening, function of ancillary staff) and the third, an item of current interest (the vocational training act, confidentiality). It is now frequently the case that one question is of the 'short notes' variety, the candidate being required to write briefly on perhaps three topics. The three topics may be as disparate as dextropropoxyphene, age–sex registers and seborrhoeic dermatitis, and wide areas of the candidate's knowledge can be tested in this way.

The traditional essay paper lasts one and a half hours and each of the three questions must be answered. As each answer is potentially worth the same number of marks it is foolhardy for the candidate to give more weight to one than another, and an overall pass mark is far more likely to be obtained by answering three questions moderately well than by answering one brilliantly, one fairly well and one not at all. However much you may feel you know about a subject, do not be tempted to continue writing until you have said it all. Allot 30 minutes to each question and stick rigidly to your time limit. Even if you are a potential Nobel prize winner, the examiner will have only a certain number of marks which he is able to award in return for your efforts in answering one question.

Having allotted 30 minutes to each question, it is wise to divide that time further so that 5 minutes are spent planning, 20 minutes writing, and 5 minutes reading over each answer. Before you begin, make sure that you have read the question thoroughly and that you understand what the examiner requires. Do not be tempted to invent a question of your own, which can lead to disaster, or to reproduce word for word an answer to a question which bears some resemblance to that with which you are now presented. Instead, use the 'building blocks' of knowledge you possess to construct the answer sought.

Spend the first five minutes collecting your thoughts and making brief notes (which can later be crossed out) on the areas you wish to cover and the main headings you will use. This is the bare bones of your essay. The next 20 minutes will be spent on building on these notes to produce the essay itself which should be logical in sequence, practical and relevant in content, and clear and succinct in presentation. Make matters easier for both the examiner and yourself by writing legibly, spacing your answer attractively, using headings liberally and underlining headings and important points where necessary. Always begin your answer with a brief introduction and end with a conclusion. Use brief sentences and write in paragraphs and sub-paragraphs. Do not forget that reasonable spelling and syntax will make a favourable impression upon the examiner — it is usual for a few extra marks to be allotted for lucidity and presentation.

Above all, do not underestimate the importance of the traditional essay question. Devote time and thought to its preparation and it will pay valuable dividends. Give ample consideration to topics which are likely to appear — this is one part of the MRCGP examination in which this approach can be successful — and make sure that you read the relevant material, be it textbooks, journals, newspapers or government reports. Then make the best of the knowledge you have acquired by presenting it with clarity, logic and style.

Three Sample Answers

It is difficult to make points clearly about what constitutes a 'good' TEQ answer and so we are going to illustrate what we mean by letting you read and mark 3 sample answers to the same question viz:

Question

What factors govern your use and choice of antibiotic in the management of acute lower respiratory infections in general practice?

Instructions

First draft out your own answer to this question. Try to decide a rough marking schedule. Then when you are clear about the structure and the rough marking schedule you wish to use, look at our sample marking schedule on the next page. Use it to give your own answer a definite set of marks, then read answers 1, 2 and 3 and see how you would assess these performances.

Our hope is that a thoughtful consideration of the strengths and weaknesses of these sample answers will give you many helpful hints on how to avoid answering badly yourself.

Question

What factors govern your use and choice of antibiotic in the management of acute lower respiratory infections in general practice?

Answer

1 Definition of criteria for diagnosis
  Discussion of whether to prescribe or not   1 mark

2 Quality of the illness
  - Severity and rate of progress
  - Systemic or localised   2 marks

3 Characteristics of the patient
  - Age, sex, previous health
  - Present health, e.g. pregnancy, history of allergy or idiosyncrasy
  - Other current treatment, e.g. steroids, estimate of patient
    reliability (compliance)   2 marks

4 Choice of antibiotic
  - Bacteriological basis, e.g. real or assumed
  - Sensitivities of organisms
  - Formulation, dose and frequency of antibiotic
  - Possible contraindications
  - Cost   4 marks

To be awarded at discretion of examiner: 1 mark

There are numerous factors which would influence the choice of antibiotic in the management of acute lower respiratory infection. It must always be remembered that most often a combination of some or several of these factors influences one's decision.

Age of Patient

Very young — most likely to be a lobar or bronchopneumonia.

Older children and adult — less likely to develop complications if otherwise well and can possibly be dealt with at first by simple supportive methods.

Elderly — many older people have other illnesses — chronic bronchitis, cardiac disease, also renal disease. A lower respiratory infection in this group would be life endangering and it is probably wise to start immediately with antibiotics.

Previous History

A child or adult who has a previous history of repeated upper and lower respiratory infections should receive antibiotics. Also cases of rheumatic heart disease and children with bronchospasm (spastic bronchitis).

Congenital heart disease — especially of the cyanotic variety.

The Attack – The Examination – The Findings

When examined the *clinical findings* are the best guide to the use of antibiotics — always considering other factors.

If clinically there is evidence of invasive disease of the lung, i.e. bronchial breathing, crepitations, consolidation, the clinical finding should suggest the use of antibiotics.

If there is evidence of a *pleural effusion* then tuberculosis should be suspected and confirmed before specific treatment is started.

If clinically there are no findings and the patient appears not too ill, cough mixtures and antipyretics can be given. A lot of lower respiratory infections are due to virus infections and antibiotics have no effect. A sputum culture may reveal specific organisms and indicate the correct antibiotic to be used.

If the illness continues, the position might have to be reassessed as viral infections often have secondary bacterial infections superimposed. Clinical examination, aided by x-rays and blood examinations could help. C-eosinophilia in Loeffler's syndrome or low white cell count with a high sedimentation rate in tuberculosis.

Social Factors

These play a very important part in deciding whether to hold back antibiotics. Several racial groups have heard about the wonders of antibiotics in respiratory and other illnesses and often demand antibiotics for any illness with a fever. The practitioner often has a difficult decision to make in such cases.

Long distances between the patient's home and the surgery may make it difficult for repeat visits, especially in a busy practice or where patients cannot afford the expense of travelling backwards and forwards to the surgery.

TEQ
SAMPLE ANSWER 2

The question is two-fold: what factors govern the use of an antibiotic, and what factors govern the choice of an antibiotic in acute lower respiratory infections?

When faced with the acute respiratory infection in a child, an adult or an elderly person, the general practitioner must decide if the infection is one that is going to respond to antibiotics. Antibiotics have no place in the treatment of viral pneumonias but can be used to prevent a superadded bacterial infection. Ideally all infections should be proved to be bacterial by taking sputa for culture of the organism and sensitivity but this is not always practicable and in a busy general practice situation it is not feasible.

The patient should certainly be thoroughly examined, and pulmonary consolidation or adventitious sounds may indicate a pulmonary infection. Diagnosis could be supported by a white cell count and ESR and a chest x-ray may show the pulmonary inflammation.

So it may be decided that an antibiotic is necessary. Next, the most suitable antibiotic should be chosen and one should always think of cost effectiveness. Do not give an expensive antibiotic when an equally effective cheaper one will do. Without waiting for sputum culture, one should think of the most likely infections and their response to antibiotics.

In acute pneumonia, the commonest bacterial infection would be due to the pneumococcus and the ideal choice is penicillin V. An intramuscular dose of benzyl penicillin of 1 mega unit may be given and followed by oral penicillin if the severity of the infection warrants. Oral penicillin V is still the antibiotic of choice for children and one must remember never to give tetracyclines to children and pregnant women, due to the effect on dentition. In penicillin resistant cases, erythromycin is ideal for children. Co-trimoxazole (Septrin) is also a useful but more expensive alternative.

In cases of acute or chronic bronchitis, the most likely organism is *Haemophilus influenzae* and for this, ampicillin 250 mg qds is the antibiotic of choice, or its derivatives, amoxycillin or talampicillin.

Tuberculosis is not usually considered to be an acute infection but may present as one and one should always keep this in mind particularly with immigrant populations. More detailed investigation by chest x-ray, sputum cultures and Heaf test are usually required before treatment for this condition is started and may require referral to hospital as an inpatient.

The usual treatment nowadays is initially streptomycin followed by rifampicin and isoniazid for one year.

TEQ
SAMPLE ANSWER 3

1. If the patient has been otherwise fairly fit, has a clear white sputum, a non-purulent, non-productive cough and the chest sounds clear then usually this patient does not require an antibiotic.

2. In an elderly patient I would sometimes give an antibiotic even in such cases when there is not a purulent productive cough.

3. Patients with a history of chronic or recurrent bronchitis will require antibiotics much sooner — even for prophylaxis — before more severe symptoms develop; likewise, patients with a history of asthma, cardiac history, diabetes mellitus, or steroid, or any other accompanying debilitating illness.

4. The choice of antibiotic is governed by the organisms it will eliminate, possible side-effects and price.

Penicillin V is often effective in acute respiratory infections although will not cover organisms such as *Haemophilus influenzae* and therefore I tend not to use it in such cases, though it is cheap.

Septrin, ampicillin and oxytetracycline are all in the cheaper range of antibiotics — tend to have few side-effects, and cover the common organisms, such as *Haemophilus,* staphylococcal and streptococcal infections.

If patients are unable to swallow tablets, all these three antibiotics can be obtained in a soluble form. Children under 10 years should not be given tetracyclines because of discoloration of the secondary dentition; likewise tetracyclines should not be given to pregnant patients because of damage to the dentition of the fetus in later years. Ampicillin is the drug of choice for pregnant women.

If a patient is allergic or sensitive to penicillin or one of the other antibiotics, this, of course, would affect one's choice.

With regard to the antibiotics listed above, ampicillin, oxytetracycline and Septrin are all broad spectrum antibiotics — unlike penicillin V — and therefore will cover a wider range of organisms. This leads to more rapid recovery of the patient and fewer consultations in the surgery.

COMMENTS ON TEQ SAMPLE ANSWERS

TP Answer 1 is good as far as it goes. Items 1, 2, 3 of the marking schedule are well covered but the second half of the question about the actual antibiotic to choose is not covered at all. Accordingly this answer is really being marked out of 6 instead of 10.

TP Answer 2 A reasonably good answer. It appreciates the question is in 2 parts but does not fully answer the first part. As item 3 of the marking schedule is not really mentioned this answer is being marked out of 8.

TP Answer 3 Covers both parts of the question but fairly superficially and misses a few essential points. Being marked out of 10, it would probably score about 6.

Time allowed — 90 minutes.
All three questions must be answered.

Q1 Discuss in detail the advice you would give to a 60-year-old overweight male smoker with persistent symptoms of reflux oesophagitis.

Q2 Write short notes on:
    A   Carpal tunnel syndrome.
    B   Lumps in the breast.

Q3 A three-month-old baby has died while asleep. What factors are known to be significant and what theories are held about cot or sudden infant death? Discuss those aspects of the problems that you would wish to explore at the initial and subsequent consultations with the affected family.

THE ANSWERS TO TEQ TEST 1 BEGIN ON PAGE 136

Time allowed – 90 minutes.
All three questions must be answered.

Q1 What is the function of a health visitor and how might her special skills and knowledge be of value in an attachment to a practice?

Q2 A 30-year-old unmarried female teacher consults you because she has been sleeping badly and wants a prescription for sleeping pills. How would you deal with this situation?

Q3 Write short notes on:
   A The risk of death from circulatory diseases in combined contraceptive pill takers.
   B Contraceptive use of depot progesterones.
   C The possible adverse effects of copper containing IUCDs.

THE ANSWERS TO TEQ TEST 2 BEGIN ON P 140

Time allowed – 90 minutes.
All three questions must be answered.

Q1 A 25-year-old secretary comes to see you after having been sent home from work with a 'severe' headache. How would you establish the probable cause and nature of the headache?
State briefly how you would manage the situation.

Q2 What are the advantages and disadvantages of breast as opposed to bottle feeding? Discuss how you might try to increase the number of maternity patients, within your practice, who will breast feed.

Q3 Write out a prescription for the following cases giving your reasons and approximate costs of the items prescibed:

A Male, 35, with PH of duodenal ulcer, has had epigastric pain and heartburn for 5 days.

B Female, 17, with sore red throat, cough, tender cervical glands and fever for 2 days.

C Male, 56, sudden painful swelling of right first metatarsophalangeal joint. Area is red, hot and very tender.

THE ANSWERS TO TEQ TEST 3 BEGIN ON P 145

TEQ
TEST 4

Time allowed − 90 minutes.
All three questions must be answered.

Q1 The mother of a two-month-old baby comes to ask your advice about whooping cough vaccination. What information would you give her to help her make up her mind? What are the contraindications to this vaccination?

Q2 The rates of home visiting by general practitioners vary. Discuss factors which may influence these rates.

Q3 Write short notes on the nature, presentation and management of:
A   Tennis elbow
B   Wax in the ear.
C   Spontaneous pneumothorax.

THE ANSWERS TO TEQ TEST 4 BEGIN ON P 150

TEST 1 ANSWERS

Q1   Discuss in detail the advice you would give to a 60-year-old overweight male smoker with persistent symptoms of reflux oesophagitis.

A1   **1. *Introduction***

Persisting symptoms mean problem must be taken seriously to prevent progression to ulceration and stricture.

Reassure patient that he does not have heart disease and that though his condition has a high nuisance value it is unlikely to become serious provided he follows your advice. Correcting superimposed anxiety should increase pain threshold.   2 marks

2. *Advice*

Based on knowledge of the behaviour of the lower oesophageal sphincter (the second line of approach is the use of drugs which has *not* been asked for in the question).

Stop smoking – cigarette smoking reduces the lower oesophageal sphincter pressure which then allows reflux, especially when smoking after a meal. Forceful advice from GP may help patient to stop.   1 mark

Lose weight – not certain why this helps. Possibly from reduction in rich, fatty meals and also the size of meals. Diet sheets/supervision by practice nurse.   1 mark

Diet – fatty meals, xanthine containing foods (coffee, chocolate), alcohol and carminatives (peppermint) decrease lower oeseophageal sphincter pressure and should be avoided.

Acid fruit drinks may aggravate pain from oesophagitis.   1 mark

Size of meals – symptoms of reflux are often worse after large meals so best avoided.   1 mark

Posture – reflux is less likely when patient is erect and when gravity assists oesophageal clearing. Avoid stooping or bending, eating in low chairs, wearing tight undergarments and belts.   1 mark

Sleeping – symptoms at night may be avoided by patient raising head of bed on bricks or blocks by 8 to 11 inches. This gives great benefit and markedly reduces both duration and frequency of reflux. Pillows do not provide an effective alternative.

Sleeping on the left side or in the prone position may affect anatomical relationship of gastro-oesophageal junction and decrease symptoms.   1 mark

3. *Conclusion*

Important to take the time to give adequate explanation and reassurance.

Relevant advice is essential for successful management.

Written instructions – diet and anti-smoking handouts may help increase compliance.

Follow up will allow further discussion and explanation and monitoring of progress.

2 marks

Q2 Write short notes on:
   A   Carpal tunnel syndrome.
   B   Lumps in the breast.

A1   A. Carpal Tunnel Syndrome

1. *Introduction*

Intermittent median neuritis due to pressure beneath flexor retinaculum.

Females 8: males 1.

Frequently bilateral.

Peak age 40 to 50 years.

May be due to pregnancy, myxoedema, rheumatoid arthritis.   2 marks

2. *Characteristics*

Pain, paraesthesiae, hypoaesthesia ± numbness in thumb, index finger, middle finger and lateral half of ring finger (sensory). Possible wasting of thenar eminence (motor).

Usually at night and recurrent.

Fingers swollen, hand heavy.

Relieved by hanging arm or walking about.

Worsened by forced palmar flexion, tapping over carpal tunnel, venous compression (sphygmo), increased use of hand/arm.   2 marks

3. *Treatment*

Analgesics.

Diuretics.

Cock up splint at night.

Steroid injections.

Operation to divide flexor retinaculum.   1 mark

B. Lumps in the Breast

1. *Introduction*

Painless lump found in breast is commonest mode of presentation of benign and malignant lesions. Source of great anxiety to women.

May be multiple/generalised, cystic or solid.   1 mark

2. *Characteristics*

Mastitis — physiological, e.g. neonatal, puberty.
           — chronic fibroadenotic   — common, peak age 30 to 50 years
                                — due to hormone imbalance
                                — benign
                                — tender breast tissue
                                — cyclical, usually bilateral
                                — usually resolves in time
                                — treat by reassuring and re-examining mid-cycle. Possible premenstrual diuretics or progesterone or 'pill'.
                                — if in doubt refer.   1 mark

Cystic — may be part of 'mastitis'
         — may be aspirated with fluid for cytology.   0.5 marks

Solid — fibroadenoma   — under 30
                           — firm, painless, mobile lump
                           — no glands in axilla
                           — refer for excision.   1 mark

      — carcinoma   — common, 5 per cent of women, 11,000 deaths/year
                           — family history
                           — cardinal sign is attachment to other structures
                           — glands may be hard or enlarged
                           — refer for biopsy/treatment   1 mark

3. *Investigation/Diagnosis*

Screening — ?value (HIP study).
Self-examination, clinical examination, mammography.   0.5 marks

Q3 A three-month-old baby has died while asleep. What factors are known to be significant and what theories are held about cot or sudden infant death? Discuss those aspects of the problem that you would wish to explore at the initial and subsequent consultations with the affected family.

A3 ## 1. *Factors*

Increased incidence in babies who are
— males
— artificially fed
— slow weight gain
— poor birth weight
— lower social classes

Before death — 1/3 babies serious illness
— 1/3 babies mild/nonspecific illness
— 1/3 babies healthy (?gently battered)

Viruses may well be implicated.   2 marks

2. *Theories*

Immunological incompetence in response to infection.

Anaphylaxis.

Hypernatraemia.

Arrhythmias

Airway obstruction during muscular relaxation in the REM phase of sleep.

GOK (God only knows!).

Undoubtedly there is no one cause for all cases.   2 marks

3. *Initial Interview*

Family's reaction will be shock/disbelief (exaggerated grief reaction).

Sympathetically explain what has happened.

Stress no suspicion of parental neglect.

Explain no definite cause known.

Explain *must* be postmortem as 'sudden' death.

Bear in mind possibility of introducing parents to similarly affected families (via the
Foundation for the Study of Infant Deaths).   3 marks

4. *Intermediate Interview* (*within a few days or so*)

Variable number of sessions will be needed with how?, why?, etc. questions having
to be answered and reanswered.

Constant reassurance will be needed.

Hostility against GP, hospital, other parent should be ventilated and explored.

Community tendency to blame the parents for neglect should also be considered.

Siblings should not be forgotten as they will feel insecure and may wonder if they too will die.   2 marks

5. *Late Interview*

Further discussion of aetiology, etc.

If more children wanted then explain recurrence rate is 4 to 7 times greater than for general population.

Marriage and sexual stresses caused by the death may need to be explored.   1 mark

TEQ
TEST 2

TEST 2 ANSWERS

Q1   What is the function of a health visitor and how might her special skills and knowledge be of value in an attachment to a practice?

A1   1. *Introduction*

Either SRN with part one midwifery and one year HV certificate at university *or* integrated 4 year university/nursing course.
Employed by AHA, not GP, and while will work with him and his patients is under the control of her own hierarchy on the community health side.   1 mark

2. *Function*

Provides health education and social advice to families and individuals in the community.   1 mark

—   maternal care — antenatal clinics and follow-up of non-attenders
                  — advice re diet/exercise, etc.
                  — mothercraft/relaxation classes   1 mark

— child care — obligation to visit all children from 0 to 5 years for whom she is responsible (was statutory duty until 1974)
   — well baby/development clinics
   — immunisation
   — home visiting   1 mark

— welfare of aged — assessment of overall needs and assistance in any regular visiting programme   0.5 marks

— mental health — early observation and help   0.5 marks

— health education   0.5 marks

— care of certain minor illnesses giving social support and health education
                                                                        0.5 marks

3. *Value to Practice*

General purpose family medicosocial worker who can handle many of the less complicated social problems, especially those with some medical content.

Can identify problem families/family problems at an early stage.

Can cooperate in joint ventures — development/immunisation clinics, screeening programmes, health education.

Can liaise with social workers in 'at risk' cases.

Patients benefit from HV attached to practice
— all problems handled in one place
— primary care team concept fostered
— easy communication of their problems between HV/GP.   4 marks

Q2   A 30-year-old unmarried female teacher consults you because she has been sleeping badly and wants a prescription for sleeping pills. How would you deal with this situation?

A2   1. *Introduction*

Important to relate care to knowledge of patient

   Previous personal knowledge of her family history

   Work history

   Recent stresses, etc.

PH in records   — depression
                 — anxiety
                 — overdosage
                 — physical ills.   2 marks

2. *Assessment of Presenting Symptom*

Why sleeping badly?
- ?   reactive to obvious stresses/strains
  - personal life (unmarried at 30)
  - work (teacher)
- ?   part of depressive condition
- ?   associated with physical illness
  - check for symptoms/signs, e.g. thyrotoxicosis, UTI, URTI.

What pattern of sleep disturbance?
- ?   can't get off
- ?   restlessness
- ?   dreams
- ?   early morning waking   2 marks

3. *Making a Diagnosis*

Diagnosis must be made before prescribing sleeping pills.

Subsequent management will depend on diagnosis.

Most likely to be depression/anxiety.   1.5 marks

4. *Management*

Explain nature of condition to patient.

Consider whether treatment with antidepressant needed.

Discuss possible ways of relaxation and aiding natural sleep,
i.e. hot baths, sweet music, book, warm bed, hot drink, sex.

If it seems likely that a hypnotic may be necessary then prescribe for short period
to tide over immediate crisis only.   3 marks

5. *Which Hypnotic?*

If secondary to depression then tricyclic with sedative effect, e.g.
amitryptyline nocte.

If no depression then a suitable benzodiazepine for one week only.

See in one week.   1.5 marks

6. *Summary*

Sleep disturbance is a symptom of an underlying condition.

Make diagnosis before prescription.

Most likely 'depression—anxiety'.

Q3 Write short notes on:
A   The risk of death from circulatory diseases in combined contraceptive pill takers.
B   Contraceptive use of depot progestogens.
C   The possible adverse effects of copper containing IUCDs.

A3 **A**

1. *Introduction*

Deaths from myocardial infarction, malignant hypertension and cerebral thrombosis appear to occur with an overall excess mortality of about 1 per 5000 users of the pill per year.   1 mark

Topic is of immense interest to the media and GP may be asked by patient for his assessment of the risks.

2. *Risk of Death*

Strongly related to age (marked increase once over age of 35).

Strongly related to cigarette smoking (for all risks this by itself is more dangerous than the pill but does appear to act synergistically with the pill).

Related to obesity
    — diabetes mellitus
    — hypertension
    — familial hyperlipidaemia.

May be related to duration of use.   2 marks

3. *Summary*

Careful screening and follow up of women on pill for these risk factors may help to decrease incidence.   1 mark

B

1. *Introduction*

Only licensed in GB for use in women post-rubella vaccination or waiting for their husband's vasectomy to become effective. 1 mark

2. *Depot Progestogens*

Depo-provera (depomethoxyprogesterone acetate) 150 mg i.m. is effective for three months.

Inhibits ovulation and is as effective as combined pill.

Irregular bleeding and amenorrhoea are the most common side-effects.

Does not seem to delay significantly return of fertility after injections are discontinued. 2 marks

C

Possible IUCD Adverse Effects

Pregnancy
— in about 2 per cent per year
— increased spontaneous and septic abortion rate
— no increase in still birth or congenital abnormality rate
— possible ectopic site must be considered.

Infection
— increased risk of pelvic inflammatory disease with possible future infertility
— most significant in nulliparous patients.

Uterine bleeding and pain — about 10 per cent of women will have IUCD removed because of this, mostly in first year of use.

Expulsion — 10 per cent expelled, mainly in first year of use.

Perforation — rare but potentially serious effect of insertion.

Copper allergy — although theoretically possible does not seem to occur.

3 marks

TEST 3 ANSWERS

Q1 A 25-year-old secretary comes to see you after having been sent home from work with a 'severe' headache. How would you establish the probable cause and nature of the headache?
State briefly how you would manage the situation.

A1 ## 1. *Probabilities*

Highly likely	— tension headache (± anxiety/depression)	may be difficult to differentiate
	— migraine	
	— virus infection.	
Less likely	— sinusitis	
	— cervical spondylosis.	
Highly unlikely	— meningitis	
	— acute glaucoma	
	— subarachnoid haemorrhage	
	— brain tumour	
	— malignant hypertension.	2 marks

2. *Initial Impression*

Previous knowledge of patient

? Looks ill, feverish, in pain.   1 mark

3. *History*

Frequency, duration, site, quality (dull, throbbing, bursting, tight band, etc.).
Radiation.

Time of onset — waking, evening, weekend, premenstrual, etc.

Precipitating factors — foods, chocolate, alcohol, stress, RTA (whiplash), recent illness/URTI, drugs, etc.

Relieving factors — analgesics, rest, dark room, etc.

Aggravating factors — bending down, bright light, moving, coughing, neck movements, etc.

145

Associated features — sleep, appetite, mood, personality change, nausea, vomiting, vertigo, visual aura, photophobia, etc.

Family history.   2.5 marks

4. *Examination*

Temperature, pulse, BP.

Eyes — pupils, nystagmus, fundi, pressure.

Local tenderness — face
                   — temporomandibular joint
                   — teeth
                   — scalp (temporal arteries)
                   — neck.

Movement of cervical spine/neck stiffness.

CNS or other systems only if indicated.   1.5 marks

5. *Management*

General — explanation, reassurance, certificate.

Tension headache— counselling
                — analgesics p.r.n.
                — ? tranquillisers/antidepressants.

Migraine   — keep diary/avoid trigger factors
                — analgesics/anti-emetics
                — ergotamine and appropriate advice
                — ?preventative drugs (clonidine, beta blockers).

Toxic headache — general measures
                — analgesics
                — antibiotics if indicated.

Cervical headache— rest, analgesics
                — traction
                — collar.

Subarachnoid

Meningitis

Glaucoma   admit to hospital

Malignant hypertension

Space occupying lesion   3 marks

Q2 What are the advantages and disadvantages of breast as opposed to bottle feeding? Discuss how you might try to increase the number of maternity patients, within your own practice, who will breast feed.

A2 ## 1. *Advantages*

Prevention of infection, especially gastroenteritis, but also respiratory infections, septicaemia and thrush.

Prevention of cot deaths.

Protection against food allergy/eczema.

Free, easier for mother as no preparation, designed for the baby so easily digested.

Decreases ovulation so birth spacing effect.

Possibly decreases incidence of carcinoma of the breast (evidence arguable).

Possibly increases bonding with less risk from accidental injury.

Lower incidence of — obesity
                    — intestinal obstruction due to inspissated milk
                    — dental caries
                    — tetany
                    — ulcerative colitis.   4.5 marks

2. *Disadvantages*

Drugs and other substances may cross from mother to baby.

Less freedom for mother with possible embarrassment when feeding.

Painful breasts or nipples. Possible abscess.

Loose stools give more cleaning to do.

Baby may be underfed without Mum knowing.   2.5 marks

3. *Health Education*

Ensure all partners bring subject of breast feeding up with antenatal patients and discuss any doubts they may have about it.

Ensure attached staff (health visitors, district midwives) are aware of the advantages of breast feeding and the practice policy relating to it. Ensure they bring the subject up with antenatal patients.

Liaise with local obstetric unit (especially midwives) to ensure they help practice patients who wish to breast feed.

Advise on breast care antenatally.

Posters/pamphlets displayed prominently in surgery.

Articles in local press/talks to patient groups/any other advertising measures.

3 marks

Q3 Write out a prescription for the following cases giving your reasons and approximate costs of the items prescribed:

A Male, 35, with PH of duodenal ulcer, has had epigastric pain and heartburn for 5 days.

B Female, 17, with sore red throat, cough, tender cervical glands and fever for 2 days.

C Male, 56, sudden painful swelling of right first metatarsophalangeal joint. Area is red, hot and very tender.

A3 A

Likely Diagnosis

Flare-up of old DU and probably gastro-oesophageal reflux.   0.5 marks

Prescription

Tabs Magnesium trisilicate compound, two oral four-hourly. — 70   1 mark

Reasons   — short duration of attack
       — may settle with antacids
       — advise on frequent small meals
       — review in one week.   1.5 marks

Cost

Approx 40 to 45p (Drug Tariff, 1980 DHSS)   0.5 mark
(NB Any appropriate antacid with correct cost will do for answer).

B

Likely Diagnosis

Acute viral pharyngitis with cervical adenitis.   0.5 marks

May be acute tonsillitis but if so is still likely to be viral (less than 40 per cent are due to streps).   1 mark

Prescription

None necessary.

Advise — you have a virus infection
  — it will take four to five days to recover
  — take plenty of fluids
  — take two aspirins or paracetamols four-hourly
  — stay off work (give certificate)
  — stay in bed if you feel 'bad'.
                                                          2 marks

Cost

Nil. If prescribe soluble aspirin then cost about 15p for 30.

C

Likely Diagnosis

Acute gout.   0.5 mark

Prescription

Phenylbutazone 100 mg, one tablet two-hourly for first 12 hours then one tablet four-hourly until pain controlled. — 50

Acute gout can be controlled by
  — phenylbutazone
  — indomethacin
  — corticosteroids
  — colchicine
  — other anti-inflammatory drugs.

Choice of phenylbutazone (or indomethacin) depends on doctor's familiarity with drug and knowledge of its safety.

Reason for 50 tablets is for him to keep in case of further attacks.

May require long-term management with allopurinol.   2 marks

Cost

Approx 20p for phenylbutazone.   0.5 mark

TEST 4 ANSWERS

Q1 The mother of a two-month-old baby comes to ask your advice about whooping cough vaccination. What information would you give her to help her make up her mind? What are the contraindications to this vaccination?

A1 ## 1. *Introduction*

This is the vaccination which worries most parents. Since the concern over its safety was voiced in 1974 the percentage of children vaccinated, under two years, has dropped from 78 per cent to 31 per cent and there has been a major rise in the incidence of whooping cough (74,000 cases in 1977 to 1978).   0.5 marks

2. *Facts to Present*

Whooping cough remains a serious disease causing death as well as an unknown number of cases of brain and lung damage.   1 mark

Newborn babies have little or no immunity and the disease is most serious in the first year of life.   0.5 mark

Medical treatment is ineffective with no antibiotic altering the clinical course and no cough medicine affecting the cough.   1 mark

10 per cent of children below the age of two with whooping cough have to be admitted to hospital.   0.5 mark

Vaccination is about 90 per cent effective.   0.5 mark

Minor reactions to vaccination occur in about 10 per cent of children and resolve within 24 to 48 hours.   0.5 marks

About 8 per cent of all children have a fit at some stage in childhood. The fever provoked by pertussis vaccination may produce a benign febrile convulsion. There is little evidence that fits are caused by the vaccine itself.   1 mark

Very occasionally vaccination may cause serious brain damage. It is nearly impossible to define the actual risk but about 1 in 100,000 (as for measles) would seem a fair guess. If damage is going to occur then it will probably occur within 24 hours of the vaccination being given.   1 mark

All immunisations carry some risks.   0.5 marks

3. Contraindications

Genuine contraindications are few and even they are arguable. As long as the DHSS advises that some condition is a contraindication then, whatever the merits of their argument, for medicolegal reasons the vaccine should not be given.   1 mark

History of fits in the child or close family — advised by the DHSS though specifically stated as not being a contraindication by the American authorities.   0.5 marks

Pre-existing abnormality of the brain or nervous system — the evidence that this might increase the risk is very slender.   0.5 marks

Severe reaction to a previous dose of vaccine may be followed by grave consequences if second injection given.   0.5 marks

Child with any infection — this does not increase the likelihood of vaccine reaction but some sequelae of the infection (e.g. meningitis, encephalitis) may be blamed on the vaccine.   0.5 marks

Q2 The rates of home visiting by general practitioners vary. Discuss factors which may influence these rates.

A2 ## 1. Introduction

Rates range by 20 fold from 0.1 to 2 per patient per year (quote Trends in General Practice; Second Morbidity Survey 1970–71 OPGS/RCGP).

Changing attitudes to home visiting
  — by public — more prepared and able to attend surgery.
  — by GPs — less prepared to visit because of time, petrol, etc.

Refer to customs in other countries
  — USA/Canada — nil visits
  — USSR — lots of visits
  — France — lots of visits.

Pros and cons of visiting.   1.5 marks

2. The Practice

Practice policies relating to visiting
  — appointment system
  — on call duties
  — practice transport services
  — use of ancillaries
  — decision on value of social visits.

Geography
- distance and time factors
- petrol costs
- communications — percentage of patients on telephone
            — public transport systems.

Health team
- who else does visiting and should they do more.

Other duties
- hospital work
- private work.   2.5 marks

3. *The Patients*

Expectations — customs and traditions of area.

Age/sex distribution — more visits for very old and very young.

Social class.

Transport — how many patients with access to cars.

Morbidity/chronic illness.

Family support available for elderly.   2.5 marks

4. *Morbidity*

Acute illness — visiting increased especially if manage myocardial infarcts, etc. at home.

Chronic illness/disabled — social visiting by whom and how often.

Home deliveries — least often needed but lot of early discharges needing P/N follow up.

Dying at home — common reason for frequent regular visits.   1 mark

5. *General Practitioner*

Age — older GPs visit more than young GPs.

List size — paradoxically, the higher the list, the lower the visiting rate.

Length of time in practice — does this affect visiting rates?   1 mark

6. *Summary*

Pros — see home circumstances
      — cement GP/patient relations
      — prevent elderly home accidents.

Cons — wasteful of time.
       — lack facilities for proper examination/investigation
       — rarely necessary on medical grounds
       — social visits better done by nurses   1.5 marks

Q3 Write short notes on the nature, presentation and management of
   A   Tennis elbow
   B   Wax in the ear
   C   Spontaneous pneumothorax

A3 A. Tennis Elbow

What is it?

Epicondylitis of lateral epicondyle of humerus, at site of muscle insertion.

Rare in tennis players.

Common in housewives, DIY men, business men with bags.

Tends to recur.

Resolves given time.   1.5 marks

Presentation

Pain at site, i.e. external elbow.

Worse on lifting teapot, shaking hands, etc.

Localised tenderness.   0.5 marks

Management

Leave to resolve naturally if not too painful or inject local corticosteroid/local anaesthetic.

Inject into tender area   1 ml lignocaine 1 per cent
                         1 ml (40 mg) methylprednisolone

Tell patient pain will be worse for a few hours then will resolve in 48 hours.

Come again if recurs.   1 mark

B. Ear Wax

What is it?

Natural secretion of external meatal glands that serves as a lubricant and protectant.

Problems arise only if it accumulates and causes deafness or leads to otitis externa.   0.5 marks

Presentation

Deafness   — progressive or sudden
                — often worse after night lying on deaf ear side.

Often PH.

Otitis externa.   1 mark

Management

Removal.

If wax soft then syringe but if hard soften with olive oil, etc. for few days.

Syringing   — reassure patient
                — cover with towel
                — kidney dish to catch water
                — pull pinna back to straighten meatus
                — aim syringe nozzle forwards and upwards
                — gentle bursts warm water
                — examine ear when finished.

Possible complications — impacted wax
                — injury to external meatus
                — injury to drum
                — physiological vertigo
                — cough (auriculotemporal nerve stimulus).   2 marks

C. Spontaneous Pneumothorax

What is it?

Sudden deflation of lung due to rupture of bulla on lung surface giving air entry into pleural space and loss of negative pressure.
NB — tension pneumothorax is dangerous
    — pneumothorax in asthma may be bilateral and dangerous
    — pyopneumothorax may occur in staph. pneumonia.

Usually in tall thin men.

May recur.   1.5 marks

Presentation

Sudden pain/discomfort on one side of chest.

Difficulty breathing.

Irritating cough.

Hyper-resonance and absent air entry.

Confirm by x-ray of chest.   1 mark

Management

Think of possibility.

Examine chest.

Confirm by chest x-ray.

Either   — wait for slow natural recovery
         — admit for removal of air to expand lung.

Recurrence possible.   1 mark

THE ORALS

.

About four weeks after the candidates have sat for the papers, 16 out of each 20 will be invited to present themselves for oral examination in Edinburgh or London. The day and venue will be known in advance. Candidates are forewarned at the time of the papers and may arrange alternative times. Finally, 11 or 12 of each original 20 will pass the two oral examinations to become members of the Royal College of General Practitioners.

Young and vocationally trained doctors have a greater chance of passing than those not so fortunately endowed. Indeed, it is this indisputable statistic which has given rise to some criticism of the whole examination. So much so, that it is now very probable that the examination itself will be restructured in the near future to meet the objections raised by its critics. Such a prospect does not, however, help candidates intending to sit the examination as it is currently structured. This chapter, therefore, is directed towards assisting candidates to meet the existing challenge of the *viva voce*.

The young vocationally trained doctor should do well where factual recall is the major requirement and the more mature, experienced doctor should do well where problem solving and case management are the chief features of the test. For this reason the structure of the oral examination will be described in some detail. Long experience of preparing candidates for this examination has shown that familiarity with the setting and content of the examination helps to allay anxieties which so often impair a candidate's performance to a degree which may, quite unjustly, jeopardise the final result.

The Log Diary is the basis of the first oral and the Problem Solving is the basis of the second. Each oral is conducted by two examiners, neither of whom will have any information about the marks scored by the candidates in the written papers, nor will the second pair of examiners know the marks scored in the first oral.

The Log Diary (or 1st oral), an original College invention, comes from the candidate's own practice and includes 50 of his own consecutive cases.

The problem solving (or 2nd oral) is based on the examiners' own practice experiences and they will pose questions on cases and situations that they have encountered.

'. . . . his diagnosis will be composed in *physical, psychological and social terms. He will intervene educationally, preventatively and therapeutically to promote his patient's health.'* (RCGP job definition.)

The oral examiners approach the candidate assuming that he already possesses a minimum level of clinical factual knowledge as demonstrated by his having passed the written papers. They seek to test his *knowledge, skills* and *attitudes* in as many situations as is possible in the time allowed (50 to 55 minutes), but they recognise that the absence of real patients and the artificiality

157

of the situation may militate against the candidate demonstrating his full potential as a good general practitioner.

The candidate should accept the examiners as peers, as experienced general practitioners conscious of the privilege accorded them by the very presence of the volunteer sitting opposite them, and not as expendable evils or ogres! Unbelievable as it may sound, the College examiners are as reasonable and decent a body of people as you would find in any other comparable group. Although taking pardonable pride in the title of examiner, they are certainly not motivated by financial gain as they are unpaid. By and large they prefer to pass rather than fail a candidate.

Each candidate then will be examined by four examiners, two pairs in each of two separate orals, for approximately half an hour in each case.

The end of the oral is signalled by a gong or bell — always welcome to the candidate and not infrequently to the examiners as well!

Nowadays, a third or even a fourth person is likely to be present at the oral examination, acting as observers assessing the examiners, but neither will take any active part in the discussions.

All the examiners take their turn in acting as such observers and are asked to comment upon and rate the performance of the *examiner*. They are not asked to give an opinion on the candidate unless an impasse develops between the individual examiners. It should be noted here that examiners have to be prepared to justify their failing of a candidate in front of a group of senior examiners (the Executive). Similarly, if there is too wide a discrepancy of marks between individual, or pairs of, examiners the matter must be discussed in detail before a final mark is agreed.

Remember that a very good mark in one oral may not be sufficient to overcome a very poor mark in the other.

The standard of the examination has risen since 1977 and the candidate can best meet this increased challenge by improving his performance at the oral examinations — but how can his performance be improved?

The fact that he has been asked to prepare a Log Diary and given a time to attend for oral examination suggests that his basic knowledge is good enough for the College. But that knowledge was presented to the examiners in writing by a cipher, an anonymous number! The candidate thus judged to be already three-fifths worthy enough to be a member of a Royal College could be a Crippen, a Palmer or a Fellow of one of the other Royal Colleges!

Note that the word 'performance' has appeared three times in the last four paragraphs.

Look again at the scene. Four or five professional men sit around a table. Two are examining a lone figure who is only trying to prove that his last eight or nine years have not been totally wasted and that his only motive is to be a competent and safe general practitioner — never mind what his patients or teachers think about him.

Another mature, possibly distinguished looking doctor is observing the two examiners, very aware of the discomforting fact that he must concentrate on what both they and the candidate are saying. At the same time he must maintain notes on the content of the questions and answers and the knowledge, attitudes and skills of the three performers which he may have to answer for to yet more examiners. Have a thought, too, for the trainee examiner who may be the other person sitting slightly outside the group and probably more nervous than the candidate lest he be asked for any opinion whatsoever.

158

From such a scenario the inescapable conclusion is that this is a sketch, albeit a serious one, for three or more players where only two possess any sort of script.

What, the candidate will ask, are the examiners seeking to find out and how will they set about it? Fortunately, there is little variation in the way the questions are put even though the content will vary depending on the reaction of the candidate and the idiosyncrasies of the examiners.

In the first oral the questions are based on what *you have written* in the Log Diary and, in the second, the problem solving oral, the questions come from the *examiner's own experience*, but the objective of each method is the same. The examiners must decide the following:

1. Is this a safe, competent doctor worthy of admission to full membership of the Royal College of General Practitioners?

2. Does this doctor inculcate confidence and trust, is he compassionate, a man of sensibility and common sense?

3. Is he well read medically?

4. Does he see his patient as an individual person rather than as an impersonal complaint or a malady?

5. Has he got a well-developed 'third ear'?

6. How skilful is he at interviewing and problem solving?

7. How quickly does he detect the major reason for the patient coming to see the doctor even if it is not the one the patient believes it to be?

Certainly it is unfortunate that manual skills in the widest sense cannot be tested in the oral examination, for there is little doubt that some of the most caring and manually skilful doctors are relatively inarticulate

and so lose out in this, as yet imperfect, test. However, it must continue until other practical ways are devised to test this vital attribute of good general practitioners.

The candidate can do a great deal to enhance his own performance. He should first of all study his appearance and his deportment and, if possible, his behaviour under simulated examination conditions. Advice on dress and grooming might be considered impertinent but attention should be paid to this for, however old-fashioned it may seem, examiners, like patients, prefer doctors to look like doctors. This is not to imply that a tall hat, striped trousers and cut-away would guarantee success! Let sobriety and good taste be the watchword while firmly eschewing extremes of hue and cut.

The candidate should seize every opportunity to subject himself to mock orals, using audio tape and, if at all possible, spend an hour or so on videotape. The latter is of great benefit so long as the candidate graciously and honestly accepts an image of himself which can be disturbing to his self esteem.

Listen carefully and concentrate on everything the examiners say, and don't hesitate to seek clarification of any obscure point. Argue your case by all means but modulate your voice and avoid stridency. Be certain that you have sufficient facts and data for your arguments. Overall, cultivate an air of competence leavened by a touch of humour and avoid brashness, undue levity and over confidence.

Silent periods earn no marks so avoid them. Refrain from damning views contrary to those held by you, and prudently allow that all disease is made up of physical, social, mental and functional components in varying proportions all requiring note, attention, assessment and possible actions.

Avoid leading the examiner to areas of

knowledge where you know yourself to be deficient and if you insist on 'digging your own grave' remember that the examiner will happily provide you with a large spade! Do not state or record (in Log Diary) that you use appliances or carry out procedures which you do not – you will be found out and suffer accordingly.

Know your emergencies or rather urgencies. Prepare a protocol from your own practice experience for all the commonly occurring illnesses and situations. Keep abreast of the latest ideas and you ought to be aware of major research projects.

Know the drugs you use yourself and know them by their BP name, their side-effects and their incompatibilities.

Present yourself in a calm state of mind by allowing yourself plenty of time.

Be optimistic because you have passed the papers and, even if you are unfortunate enough to fail to satisfy the examiners, the experience should promote that proper sense of humility so fundamental to the attainment of great wisdom and expertise by the (primary) physician.

The First Oral (Log Diary)

This is the moment when the examiners see you for the first time as a living, sentient being rather than a mere number and it is, accordingly, an important moment for you. There is little doubt that the impression gained from the initial confrontation influences the examiners for better or for worse to a much greater extent than they would care to admit.

Most doctors have experience of the same phenomenon occurring with new patients and make, or should make, allowances for the unreasonable bias which may result. The candidate, however, may presume that experienced examiners will make the same subconscious correction. Nevertheless the candidate has nothing to lose if he makes the best use possible of whatever gifts nature has bestowed upon him.

The second important feature of this oral arises from the fact that the candidate writes the scenario and it follows, therefore, that he should be able to answer questions based on statements he has made. It is essential that he remembers what he has written and that his facts are accurate.

The Log Diary (an example is given on page 163), a College innovation, is divided into two parts. The first part is confined to a description of the candidate's practice, his work load, demographic details, ancillary services and equipment available. Although relatively few marks may be given for answers based on this section, it is equally true that floundering about or manifest ignorance would unfavourably prejudice the examiners, so do the best you can and at least attempt to convey a sense of vocation and mastery of your discipline. Do not put down equipment, staff or techniques that you do not use and are not familiar with.

The second group of questions is based on the diary of the 50 consecutive cases you have listed. They need not, of course, be consecutive for you might have chosen a day when an influenza epidemic was raging which would present a very unbalanced record, however accurate.

Ensure that it is a typical record with common problems in proper proportions, and one or two unusual or interesting cases which you may be confident will be seized upon by an examiner already jaded by the tedium of common trivia. Above all, be accurate, use cases you have looked after yourself, remember what you did and update yourself on the progress up to the time of the examination.

Bring along an aide memoire of modest size, not a folder bulging with case notes or a tome the size of a family bible! You may, however, record more than the name, age, sex and diagnosis, for there is no reason why you should not record outstanding details of investigations and treatment, especially those facts you might have difficulty remembering. You should give the impression that you know the patient personally and the family.

For ease of reference the Log Diary (or Practice Log) will be taken page by page and you should refer to the example on pages 163 to 168).

Page 1 (points 1 to 8)

Questions may be put to you on the difference between urban and rural practices.

What are the advantages or disadvantages of dispensing practices?

Have you a trainee and trainer and, if the former, should the other partners assist in the teaching? How much should he do? When should he be left on his own?

Would you prefer to work in a Health Centre? What are the objections to working in one?

Home or hospital delivery? Shared care?

What does the patient think? Which is safer? Would you deliver a baby at home if the mother refuses hospital?

Page 2 (points 9 to 15)

What special clinics do you provide?

Who runs the immunisation clinic?

Does your nurse give the injections and if so what criteria should you follow?

How much of your day does your receptionist organise?

Who deals with the difficult patient, e.g. the one who demands that her child should see a particular doctor?

How does a Practice Manager train for the job?

How does a Health Visitor achieve her qualification and what are her statutory duties? How may these be added to in the future?

What is a community nurse?

How would you cope if the social workers in your area went on strike?

When do you use an ECG — what are the disadvantages of routine ECGs?

When would you use a peak flow meter (normal values for a male adult aged 25)?

You may expect to be closely questioned on any equipment you have included in your list.

When and where do you use the laboratory facilities?

Do you know the costs of: a full blood count; LFT; serum cholesterol and triglycerides; GTT.

What do you consider would be a reasonable waiting period for a barium meal, and IVP? When are you justified in asked for an IVP? The cost of an IVP?

Page 3 (points 16 and 17)

You are likely to be questioned about appointments held outside the practice such as those in industry, hospitals, schools, nursing homes and prisons, or posts concerned with postgraduate education.

Special features of your practice should be mentioned, e.g. racial characteristics, predominant age groups, social class, industry, vandalism, housing, amenities, social services and any others you may feel need noting.

Policy on house visits and deputising services are likely. Practice protocols mentioned in Section 17 of the example would be followed up, as would the claim that the practice prescribing rate is very low and that the practice is involved in an MRC hypertension trial.

Page 4

Questions are unlikely unless anomalies are evident such as the fact that no repeat home visits are listed in the sample.

Pages 5 and 6

The list of cases given covers a wide spectrum and splendidly illustrates the advice given earlier. The only problem the examiners will have is choosing from such a range.

From the candidate's point of view it could be said with some truth that he has made a rod for his own back and this would certainly be the case if he has not fully briefed himself on every patient. It follows that weaker, less confident candidates should select their cases with great care and, without hesitation, exclude those with rare, bizarre or exotic features. It is also true that any one or more of these cases may be used as a convenient starting point for a searching oral examination on a wide range of everyday clinical subjects.

On days prior to the oral exam you should go over each case a few times at your leisure and check, improve and amend your own aide memoire notes as and when necessary.

After 25 to 30 minutes of this you are reprieved, so to speak, by the bell, but before you take your leave of the examiners they will hand you a piece of paper on which one of them will have recorded the subjects covered by them. This you give to the next examiners, thereby ensuring that you are not asked the same questions again. Nor are you likely to be asked the questions put to you in the papers.

PRACTICE LOG

Analysis of Work Load and Practice Organisation

NAME. . .Mark Richard Collins. . . . .

ADDRESS. . .The Health Centre, Medwell, Surrey . . . .

The following analysis will assist the Panel of Examiners to assess you in your examination performance.

The audit will not in itself attract any marks but will help the examiners to enquire into your knowledge of practice organisation and discuss with you the patients you have seen recently.

Please complete pages 1, 2, 3 and 4 and on pages 5 and 6 record details of fifty consecutive patients seen.

1. *Practice List Size* 21,700

2. *Your Status in the Practice* —

  Principal [X] Assistant [   ] Trainee [   ]

3. *Length of Experience in General Practice* [6 years]

4. *Number of Years in Post* [1 year]

5. *Type of Practice*

  Rural [   ] Urban [X] Mixed [   ] Dispensing [   ]

  Teaching [X]

6. *Type of Premises*

  Converted [   ] Purpose Built [   ] Health Centre [X]

7. *Total Number of Doctors in Practice*
  (Providing General Medical Services)

  Full-time Partners | 7 |
  Part-time Partners | — |
  Assistants | — |
  Trainee Assistants | 2 |

8. *Obstetric Commitment of the Practice*

Number of confinements in complete care   **13**   GP unit at

Number of confinements in shared care   **69**   local hospital.

(These figures should refer to a recent quarter for which figures are available)

9. Total number of night visits (11 p.m. − 7 a.m) made by the Candidate during the most recent complete month   **4**

10. *Appointments System*   YES / ~~NO~~   FULL / ~~PARTIAL~~

11. *Special Sessions: Specify*
    e.g.   Ante-natal Clinic
         Immunisation
         Cytology

     Immunisation Clinics x 2 . . . .

     Antenatal/Postnatal Clinic . . . .

     Family Planning Clinic . . . .

     Well Baby Clinic . . . .

12. *Staff Employed : Specify*

     Switchboard Operator
     Cleaners x 4
     Caretakers x 2

     Practice Manager . . . .

     Receptionists x 11 . . . .

     Secretaries x 2 . . . .

     Treatment Room Nurses x 5 . . . .

     Nursing Practitioners x 2

13. *Staff Attached : Specify*

     Health Visitors x 4 . . . .

     Community Nurses x 5 . . . .

     Social Worker x 1 session per week. . . . . .

     Midwives x 3 . . . .

14. *Additional Diagnostic Equipment*
    e.g. ECG, Peak Flow Meter

     ECG . . . .

     Peak Flow Meter . . . .

     Skin Testing Equipment (allergies) . . . . .

     Audiometer . . . .
     Age/Sex Register

15. *Diagnostic Facilities to which open or direct access is available : Specify*

Full Haematology, Bacteriology ....

and Clinical Chemistry. ....

X-rays except IVP's, Barium ....

meals and enemas ....

16. *Posts held outwith the Practice, e.g. Hospital Sessions*

One partner is Area Organiser for Vocational Training. ....

. . . .

. . . .

. . . .

17. *Any special Characteristics of your Practice to which you wish to draw attention, e.g. Teaching, Geographical Features, Special Features:*

A high work load practice in a designated area. Despite this and being in a new town has

national average age/sex distributions and mainly social classes 2, 3 and 4. Practice

policy for partners to do only NHS work (including teaching) and to have no outside

appointments. ....

. Well organised with system of day and night duty doctors to see emergencies and

patients who wish to be seen urgently but cannot get appointments quickly. ....

Extensive use of 2 nurse practitioners who run obesity, hypertensive check, family planning and cytology clinics and who also do ECG's and home investigations. Do check visits on elderly (identify from age/sex register and note those who have not been seen in previous 6/12 to 1 year and visit them) and follow up visits at doctor's request. Also do initial visit for rashes, gastroenteritis, flu, tonsillitis etc. where patient cannot or will not come to surgery.

Practice protocols have been thrashed out for dealing with some standard situations (newly diagnosed hypertensives, contraception, diabetes, prescribing) and for frequent review of prescribing/repeat prescriptions policy.

Nearly lowest prescribing rates for area.

Involved in MRC hypertension trial.

Do all own night and weekend work.

165

THE ORALS

TOTAL PRACTICE WORK LOAD OVER ONE WEEK

A summer week with 6 doctors and 1 trainee working. Lighter than average work load (apart from the visits which are average.)

1. *No. of patients seen by all doctors —*

	M	Tu	W	Th	F	Sat
Consulting a.m.	123	143	143	143	143	
Consulting p.m.	114	93	93	93	137	
Other surgeries or special clinics					40 A/N	
New home visits	18	8	12	10	14	
Repeat home visits						

2. *No. of Patients seen by the Candidate —*

	M	Tu	W	Th	F	Sat
Consulting a.m.	21	20	21	22	22	
Consulting p.m.	18	22		18	23	
Other surgeries or special clinics		2*			8	
New home visits	2	1	1	1	2	
Repeat home visits	—	—	—	—	—	

* coil fittings

List consecutively *fifty* patients seen during the week of the audit, *in the consulting room and on home visits* (excluding special clinics).

As the examiners will wish to explore particular cases it will be in your own interest to bring an aide memoire with you.

V = Visit
S = Surgery

Date	Patient's name or initials	Age	Sex	Main reasons for contact	V	S
16.7.79	Mark Madder	27	M	Seborrhoeic dermatitis		S
	Mary Westman	65	F	Depression/overdose follow-up		S
	Susan Evans	50	F	?fracture patella.		S
	Avril Ivy	18	F	Pill prescription/check		S
	Brenda Jones	49	F	Chronic anxiety neurosis with free floating anxiety attacks		S
	Gillian Montgomery	14	F	Vomiting		S
	Jean Bridge	22	F	Asthmatic attack. PFR = 180		S
	Andrew Evans	5	M	Catarrh — not adenoidal		S
	Jackie Montrose	15	F	Exudative tonsillitis		S
	William Vales	55	M	Night cramps in legs.		S
	Frank Stout	40	M	Vasectomy counselling.		S
	Anne De Cay	33	F	Ankylosing spondylitis. Vaginal discharge.		S
	Yvonne Saunders	17	F	Unwanted pregnancy.		S
	Jack Skinner	47	M	BP check.		S
	Veronica Green	23	F	Threatened miscarriage.		S
	John Ginman	54	M	Sore right shoulder		S
	Philip Street	18	M	Acne.		S
	Mandy Painter	10	F	Recent epistaxis.		S
	Sydney Jones	58	M	Bell's palsy.		S
	Albert Shiner	62	M	Cough/URTI		S
	Doris Sofbott	43	F	Temporal lobe epilepsy out of control recently.		S
	James Orfull	68	M	Mild CVA	V	
	Eileen Nixon	74	F	Thrombophlebitis.	V	
	Jenny Singer	2	F	Mother young with illegitimate child. Difficulties coping.		S

Date	Patient's name or initials	Age	Sex	Main reasons for contact	V	S
16.7.79 Nelly Herder		77	F	Cardiac failure — marked ankle oedema.		S
Andrew Hurter		19	M	?Glandular fever.		S
Steven Williams		5	M	Constipation with overflow soiling.		S
Josephine Crest		30	F	Pill prescription. Hay Fever.		S
Elaine Orfull		64	F	Worried re health of husband who had CVA		S
Julia Hunter		35	F	Backache (small shopkeeper & determined to work.)		S
Valerie Weston		19	F	Ringworm.		S
Edith Nightingale		57	F	Otitis externa. Anxiety neurosis.		S
Albert Pattison		60	M	Hypertension. Check BP		S
Holly Ashton		62	F	Allergic rash — contact dermatitis axilla.		S
Jane Peters		8	F	Impetigo.		S
Katherine Stalker		22	F	Divorcing husband. Unwanted pregnancy.		S
Angela Wilkinson		29	F	Diarrhoea & vomiting.		S
Martin Jeevons		20	M	Sprained ankle.		S
Colin Archer		23	M	Tonsillitis.		S
Mandy Harworth		3	F	Cystitis (dysuria & secondary enuresis)		S
Agatha Poulson		40	F	Earache — dental.		S
Ruby Rightwich		48	F	Newly diagnosed angina. On betablockers.		S
Josephine Stevens		28	F	Advice re breast feeding.		S
Paulette Chalmers		20	F	Trying to get certificate for off work on very tenuous grounds.		S
Sam Heifer		4	M	Fever. No obvious cause.		S
Amanda Thomas		28	F	Progestogen only pill (breast feeding).		S
Tom Bennett		31	M	Hiatus hernia.		S
Christine English		21	F	Confirmation of pregnancy.		S
Frederick Hammond		42	M	Tennis elbow.		S
Louise Thornton		3	F	Squinting intermittently.		S

The Second Oral (Problem Solving)

In the problem solving oral there are two examiners working as a pair who decide on the sequence and the nature of the questions before the candidate appears. The examiners are *not* aware of the candidate's performance (marks) in the present or in the past examinations.

The examiners are experienced general practitioners in active clinical practice. They have their own 'hobby horses', their own strengths and weaknesses, and their own prejudices. It is intended that the second member of the pair will ensure that any such prejudices that may come through with the questioning examiner do not reflect unfairly on the candidate.

All the examiners are engaged in teaching and training. Most of the examiners are trainers and many work in academic departments of general practice.

The *method* of examination is by question and answer, supplemented by photographs, practice records, ECG recordings, equipment and instruments and specimens.

The *content* of the questions tends to be on the common problems of general practice with certain special challenges and tests incorporated.

The *questions* are based on real clinical cases and situations from the examiners' practices. The presentation tends to be sequential somewhat on the lines of a problem solving MEQ.

The examples given at the end of this chapter show the types of questions and case histories that may be encountered.

The second oral examination tests:

1. *Attitudes and approach* of the examinee to the patient, family, community, his practice colleagues and local consultant.

2. *Awareness and assessment* of common clinical and psychosocial problems, including their frequency, age and sex distribution, their nature, causes, course and outcome.

3. *Management* of common clinical and psychosocial problems and situations. The candidate must have a clear understanding of his own management of these conditions and be prepared to defend his choice of treatment.

His methods do not have to be those followed by the examiners, but the examiners do seek evidence that he has thought out the process and can quote his own or other evidence to support his reasons. Candidates should pay particular attention to having clear protocols for his (or her) care of:

high blood pressure
cardiac failure
rheumatoid arthritis
peptic ulcer
terminal care
migraine
asthma
acute otitis media
acute tonsillitis
antenatal care
well child care
vaginal discharge
family planning
menopause
depression
eczema
psoriasis
warts
termination of pregnancy.

169

4. *Communication with patient and family* including health education and promotion of self-care, accessibility, appointment systems, out of hours cover and deputising services.

5. *Communication within the practice.* Be prepared to respond to questions on contacts with partners, receptionists, nurses and health visitors and on how practice policies are developed and created.

6. *Use of local resources and in particular:*
referrals to hospital
domiciliary consultants
urgent admissions
private practice
social services in general and to meet special situations.

7. *Quality checks*, that is, ways in which the examinee may assess and evaluate his (or her) own methods of work and those of his practice. Some thought should be given to measures of volume of work, to costs of care and to outcome of care.

8. *Recent trends and reports.* The examiners tend to read and study the *British Medical Journal, The Journal of the Royal College of General Practitioners, Update,* reports of Committees and Commissions and books. The examinee should go rapidly through all the issues of the above three journals published over the six months preceding the examination to note any important papers, reports or other relevant publications.

The examples that follow are those that have been used in the examination. They are set out as long cases (A), short cases (B), non-clinical (C) and run of the mill, bread-and-butter cases (D). An account of possible questions and answers are set out in (A) and (B) but questions only in (C) and (D). It is intended that readers will develop their own possible questions and answers to (C) and (D).

(A) Long Cases

Note that there are no 'live' clinical cases. There are no patients to be questioned and examined. There are no actors playing the parts of patients.

The long cases are patients of examiners who have presented them with useful topics and problems with which to test the examinees. It is important for the examinee to appreciate this and to place himself (herself) in the position of the examiner and, if necessary, to seek further information.

All the 'cases', long and short, contain some important but not too difficult clinical points in diagnosis or management that any experienced and alert practitioner would be expected to consider and act upon. There are no 'catches' or 'pitfalls' set to trap unwary candidates.

A1. A man aged 77 wearing a black patch over his left eye comes to consult you on account of increasingly severe aching pains in his neck, shoulder regions and back. These are worse on getting up. Symptoms have been present for six weeks. He is feeling unwell and appears to have lost weight.

Analysis (by examinee)

The black patch must be of significance. Male 77 with recent pains in neck and back, malaise and weight loss suggests some possible major systemic disorder. 'Possibles' are:
cancer of bronchus with secondary deposits
cancer of prostate with secondary deposits
myelomatosis
polymyalgia

The only correlation between the eye patch and the back pains are polymyalgia and past temporal arteritis which has left him with some loss of vision.

Questions (by examiner)

What possible diagnoses would you be thinking of?

How would you establish diagnosis?

How would you manage the case?

What are the likely prognosis and outcome?

Response (by examinee)

Cancers of bronchus or prostate with secondaries, myelomatosis or polymyalgia.

ESR raised ++ (over 75 to 100 mm per hour) in myelomatosis and polymyalgia.

X-rays of chest and spine to exclude neoplastic deposits.

Bence—Jones proteinuria — myelomatosis.

Electrophoresis pattern in myelomatosis.

If you decide on polymyalgia as the most likely diagnosis then you should be prepared to manage the case yourself with corticosteroids.

The response to steroids is dramatic and excellent.

Steroids may have to be continued for as long as 2 to 3 years.

Eventually the polymyalgia tends to 'burn itself out'.

A2 Mrs X is a married woman aged 34, whom you have known for 10 years. She has two children aged eight and six. Her husband had a vasectomy two years ago. She comes to consult you in some distress. Her menses are two weeks late.

Analysis (by examinee)

Mrs X is married — what is the state of the marriage?

You should know the family well after 10 years of care — the examiner should be asked of his knowledge of the family X.

Mrs X is a fertile woman.

Mr X has had a vasectomy.

There is a crisis situation — is Mrs X pregnant and, if so, by whom?

Questions (by examiner)

What do you ask Mrs X?

What immediate steps do you take?

How do you propose to manage the situation in relation to Mrs X and Mr X?

Response (by examinee)

Mrs X must be asked whether she may be pregnant and if so may the father not be her husband.

Before anything else is done or said to anyone she must have a pregnany test carried out. If it is negative it must be repeated. If positive then the following steps must be considered.

If no other man can be involved consider the possibility of a failed vasectomy with posssible medico-legal action against the surgeon.

If the father is not the husband consider: possible termination of the pregnany? should husband (Mr X) be informed and by whom?

A3 Your receptionist tells you that Mr M is on the phone requesting a home visit for his wife (aged 65) who has had pruritus vulvae for six weeks. She saw your partner a few days ago. She is no better and he his demanding that 'something must be done at once!'

171

Analysis (by examinee)

Mr M is angry — the situation must be defused.

The request for a home visit is unreasonable.

Your partner saw her a few days ago — you must consider his part.

Pruritis vulvae in a woman of 65 may have a serious underlying cause.

Questions (by examiner)

How do you respond to Mr M's request for a home visit?

Why is Mr M behaving as he is?

What may be the cause of the pruritis vulvae?

Response (by examinee)

Consider your receptionist's position; she is dealing with Mr M — she must be helped and supported.

You must agree to visit Mrs M at home and assess the situation and probably get her up to your consulting room for a full pelvic examination.

Mr M is under stress because he has been subjected to stress by his wife's discomfort. The marriage may be unsettled. You will seek information about the family history.

Possible causes of pruritus vulvae in a women of 65 are:
    diabetes mellitus
    atrophic vaginitis
    monilial vaginitis
    cancer of the cervix

(B) Short Cases

The short cases deal with apparently straightforward situations and the examinee is asked how he would manage them, based on his understanding of the various factors involved.

B1. A boy age five is brought to your morning consulting session with the following story. He awoke in the middle of the previous night with ear-ache. He cried for a while. Pain was relieved by aspirin. He appears well and undistressed. The left drum is red.

Analysis (by examinee)

Boy age five, in catarrhal child phase.

Acute otitis media with red drum.

General condition is good without fever or distress.

Questions (by examiner)

What do you tell the mother?

How do you manage the case and why?

Response (by examinee)

The nature, course and outcome of the catarrhal child syndrome should be transmitted to the mother with a period of liability to coughs, ear-aches and sore throats between four and seven years which is then grown out of.

Mother should be informed of the changed and benign state of otitis media now compared with the past.

Main point of debate is whether to use antibiotics or not and why and which ones?

Stress follow-up of child until drum and hearing return to normal.

B2   John F age 20 has just returned from a holiday to Tunisia. You see him at home because he has had a sore throat, fever and shivers for a few days.

Analysis (by examinee)

Young holiday maker probably living cheaply and rough.

Tunisia — a possible malarial area.

Symptoms are suggestive of an acute throat infection.

Questions (by examiner)

What advice would you give to persons holidaying in North Africa?

What may be wrong with John F?

How do you find out what is wrong?

How do you treat him?

Response (by examinee)

Advice to visitors to North Africa
  general advice on food, water and clothes
  antimalarial prophylaxis
  cholera, typhoid, tetanus and polio prophylaxis.

Possible malaria.

Possible streptococcal tonsillitis.

Check for malaria by thick blood smear.

Check for strep throat by swab.

Depending on diagnosis treat malaria or strep throat — have your protocols ready.

B3   Miss B aged 21 has had an itchy vaginal discharge for one week. She is on the Pill.

Analysis (by examinee)

She is on the Pill.

Itchy discharge — most likely cause is monilial vaginitis.

Miss B is likely to be promiscuous — remember to do a cervical smear.

Question (by examiner)

What are the likely causes of her discharge?

How do *you* investigate?

What treatment?

Response (by examinee)

Likely causes
  Monilia
  Trichomonas
  Gonococci
  Retained tampon
  Non-specific

High vaginal swab.

Cervical smear.

Treatment depends on cause.

(C) Non-clinical Cases

This is where topical non-clinical subjects may be put in for comment by examiners.

C1   *The new GP Charter*

What is it?

Who produced it?

What did it recommend?

What are your comments on it?

C2 *Health Centres*

Pros?

Cons?

What are your views of their future?

C3 *Out of Hours Cover*

How may cover be provided?

What are your views on deputising services?

C4 *'Nurse Practitioner'*

What is she (he)?

Where does she (he) practise?

What does she (he) do?

How do you see her (his) future?

C5 *GP Manpower*

How many GPs are there in the NHS?

How many do we need?

What studies/research could be done to find out?

(D) Bread and Butter Cases

These represent a good sample of a mixture of common situations that often come up as long and short cases.

D1 You are on call at night and you receive an urgent request to visit Mr P, age 56. 'He is fighting for his breath!'

What may it be?

What do you take with you? In your bag?

How would you make a diagnosis clinically?

How would you treat it?

D2 On a cold winter's morning Mr C, age 44, is pushing his car to get it to start. He is stricken by a dull heavy pain across the front of his chest. He staggers indoors. His wife phones you.

What do you say to her?

How do you assess his condition?

How do you manage him?

D3 Tony, age 10 months, is having convulsions. You see him at home.

How do you examine him?

What are you likely to find?

What do you do?

What do you say to the parents?

D4 How do you treat plantar warts?

D5 How do you manage tennis elbow?

D6 What is the approximate cost of a week's treatment of duodenal ulcer with:

aluminium hydroxide (35p)

Maxolon (£2)

Biogastrone (£3)

Tagamet (£5).

D7 What is the approximate cost of a week's treatment of acute urinary tract infection with:

oxytetracycline (30p)

ampicillin (£1)

Septrin (£3)

Furadantin (£4).

D8 Mrs B, age 34, develops an acute back pain whilst making beds. She comes to see you. She has had attacks before.

What is it?

What do you look for on examination?

What do you do for her?

What is the prognosis?

D9 Mrs C, age 54, comes to 'sign on' as a new patient. She is very talkative and complaining of her previous doctors. She asks for a tonic as she is so tired. In between her inconsequential chatter she tells you that she has had an operation for stomach ulcers 10 years go. She is pale.

What do you ask her?

What is the likely diagnosis?

What do you do?

D10 Miss D, age 20, is a foreign student studying English. She complains of constant occipital headaches for the past month.

She is tired and cannot concentrate. She suddenly bursts into tears.

What is likely to be wrong with her?

What questions would you ask her?

How do you help her?

D11 Rachel N's (age seven) mother tells you that Rachel has a sore mouth. On opening her mouth you notice a foul smell. Her gums are swollen and bleeding.

What is the likely diagnosis?

What questions?

What treatment? (It is 8 pm on a Sunday).

D12 What is your schedule of immunisation and how do you ensure compliance?

D13 What is POMR system?